Novel Approaches in the Treatment of Gastrointestinal and Liver Disease: a Look into the Future

John Libbey Eurotext
127, avenue de la République
92120 Montrouge
Tél. : 33 (0) 1 46 73 06 60
e-mail : contact@john-libbey-eurotext.fr
http://www.john-libbey-eurotext.fr

John Libbey and Company Ltd
Po Box 276
Eastleigh
SO50 5YS, England
Tel. : 44 (0) 23 80 65 02 08

CIC Edizioni Internazionali
Corso Trieste 42
00198 Roma, Italia
Tel. : 39 06 841 26 73

© John Libbey Eurotext, 2000
ISBN : 2-7420-0340-1

Il est interdit de reproduire intégralement ou partiellement le présent ouvrage - loi du 11 mars 1957 - sans autorisation de l'éditeur ou du Centre Français du Copyright, 6 *bis*, rue Gabriel-Laumain, 75010 Paris.

Novel Approaches in the Treatment of Gastrointestinal and Liver Disease : a Look into the Future

**Edited by
J.P. Galmiche**

Postgraduate Course 2000
Nantes, June 30

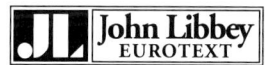

Contents

I

New targets in gastrointestinal motility disorders
J. Tack 3

Gastrointestinal-safe anti-inflammatory therapy: is it possible?
C. Scarpignato, I. Pelosini 9

Strategies against *H. pylori* infection
I. Corthésy-Theulaz, A. Blum, P. Michetti 19

II

Immunomodulation in inflammatory bowel diseases
P. Desreumaux 23

Probiotics in inflammatory bowel diseases
P. Gionchetti 29

Strategies against bacterial toxins in the gut: the case of *Clostridium difficile*
I. Just, F. Hofmann, H. Genth 33

Inhibition of intestinal secretion
M.J.G. Farthing 37

III

Multiple therapy in hepatitis C and hepatitis B
Y. Benhamou, V. Ratziu, T. Poynard 45

Gene therapy for liver diseases
J. Gournay 59

Pancreatic carcinoma: a challenge for the next century
K. Z'graggen, M. Wagner, M.W. Büchler 65

IV

Photodynamic therapy
L. Gossner 67

Laparoscopic surgery in the next century
L. R. Lundell 73

Intestinal transplantation
O. Goulet, D. Jan 77

New developments in abdominal imaging
G.N.J. Tytgat 87

List of contributors

Benhamou Y., Service d'Hépato-Gastroentérologie, Groupe Hospitalier Pitié-Salpêtrière, 47-83, boulevard de l'Hôpital, 75651 Paris Cedex 13, France.

Blum A., Division of Gastroenterology, Centre Hospitalier Universitaire Vaudois, Lausanne, Switzerland.

Büchler M.W., Department of Visceral and Transplantation Surgery, University of Bern, Inselspital, Switzerland.

Corthésy-Theulaz I., Division of Gastroenterology, Centre Hospitalier Universitaire Vaudois, Lausanne, Switzerland.

Desreumaux P., Laboratoire de Recherche sur les Maladies Inflammatoires Intestinales, CHU Lille, France.

Farthing M.J.G., Digestive Diseases Research Centre, St Bartholomew's and The Royal London School of Medicine and Dentistry, Turner Street, London, UK.

Genth M., Institut für Pharmakologie & Toxikologie der universität Freiburg, Freiburg, Germany.

Gionchetti P., Department of Internal Medicine and Gastroenterology, University of Bologna, Italy.

Gossner L., Second Medical Department, Wiesbaden Hospital, Wiesbaden, Germany.

Goulet O., Groupe de Transplantation Intestinale, Hôpital Necker-Enfants Malades, 149, rue de Sèvres, 75743 Paris Cedex 15, France.

Gournay J., Service d'Hépato-Gastroentérologie, Hôtel-Dieu, Centre Hospitalier Universitaire de Nantes, Nantes, France.

Hofmann F., Institut für Pharmakologie & Toxikologie der universität Freiburg, Hermann-Herderstr. 5, D-79104, Freiburg, Germany.

Jan D., Groupe de Transplantation Intestinale, Hôpital Necker-Enfants Malades, 149, rue de Sèvres, 75743 Paris Cedex 15, France.

Just I., Institut für Pharmakologie & Toxikologie der universität Freiburg, Hermann-Herderstr. 5, D-79104, Freiburg, Germany.

Lundell L.R., Department of Surgery, Sahlgren's University Hospital, 413 45 Gothenburg, Sweden.

Michetti P., Division of Gastroenterology, Beth Israel Deaconess Medical Center and Harvard Medical School, Boston, MA, USA.

Pelosini I., Laboratory of Clinical Pharmacology, Department of Internal Medicine, School of Medicine and Dentistry, University of Parma, Italy.

Poynard T., Service d'Hépato-Gastroentérologie, Groupe Hospitalier Pitié-Salpêtrière, 47-83, boulevard de l'Hôpital, 75651 Paris Cedex 13, France.

Ratziu V., Service d'Hépato-Gastroentérologie, Groupe Hospitalier Pitié-Salpêtrière, 47-83, boulevard de l'Hôpital, 75651 Paris Cedex 13, France.

Scarpignato C., Laboratory of Clinical Pharmacology, Department of Internal Medicine, School of Medicine and Dentistry, University of Parma, Italy ; Department of Gastroenterology and Hepatology, Faculty of Medicine, University of Nantes, France.

Tack J., Department of Internal Medicine, Division of Gastroenterology, University Hospital Gasthuisberg, University of Leuven, Herestraat 49, B-3000, Leuven, Belgium.

Tytgat G.N.J., Academic Medical Center, Department of Gastroenterology and Hepatology, Meibergdreef 9, 1105 A2, Amsterdam Zuidoost, The Netherlands.

Wagner M., Department of Visceral and Transplantation Surgery, University of Bern, Inselspital, Switzerland.

Z'graggen K., Department of Visceral and Transplantation Surgery, University of Bern, Inselspital, Switzerland.

Foreword

It is a great pleasure to host the 6th French EAGE meeting in Nantes on June 30th, 2000. It has become a tradition to hold these yearly post-graduate courses in our country just before the summer holidays. On the occasion of the new millenium, we have tried to make this meeting a very special event, and an outstanding Faculty has been invited to give lectures on the exciting topic of novel approaches to the treatment of GI and liver diseases. We are also extremely honoured that Prof G.N.J. Tytgat has agreed to chair this course which has been organised in conjunction with the French Society of Gastroenterology (SNFGE) and the Association Nationale des Gastroentérologues des Hôpitaux Généraux (ANGH).

Our original intention was not to publish the proceedings of this symposium, and speakers were only requested to provide a long abstract with 4 or 5 key references. However, many preferred to send us a full paper, and all Faculty members finally provided an excellent contribution in due time. Therefore, we decided to publish all the manuscripts as a new EAGE monograph, the 8th in the series. We are extremely grateful to Janssen-Cilag for the additional financial support that made this project feasible. As usual, our Publisher and Mrs Chantal Vezin have successfully managed the manuscripts within very short notice. We hope that you will find this monograph an interesting and useful complement to the symposium itself.

The members of the EAGE Governing Board are looking forward to seeing you soon at the next post-graduate course in Brussels on November 25th.

On behalf of the Organizing Committee,
J.P. Galmiche,
Nantes, June 15th, 2000

New targets in gastrointestinal motility disorders

Jan Tack

Department of Internal Medicine, Division of Gastroenterology, University Hospital Gasthuisberg, University of Leuven, Leuven, Belgium

Functional bowel disorders are characterized by the presence of a variety of chronic symptoms, attributed to the gastrointestinal tract, in the absence of an underlying histological, biochemical, or physiological abnormality that is able to consistently explain the symptoms [1, 2]. The pathophysiology of functional bowel disorders is not fully established, but a number of putative mechanisms have been suggested. In patients with functional bowel disorders, symptoms could originate from disordered motility, from visceral hypersensitivity, from low-grade inflammation (*e.g. Helicobacter pylori* gastritis), or from central nervous system dysfunction. Despite the fact that gastrointestinal motility disturbances have been reported to be present in patients with functional bowel disorders, their relevance and relationship to symptoms are mostly unknown. The absence of a clearly established causal relationship between symptoms and observed abnormal function has hampered the ability to target potential therapeutic approaches towards relevant specific underlying mechanisms and has lead to questioning of the motility hypothesis in functional bowel disorders [3].

Recent progress in understanding and treating functional bowel disorders was derived from two important sources. First of all, it has become clear that the so-called functional gastrointestinal syndromes are heterogeneous disorders, where distinct pathophysiological abnormalities are present in subgroups of patients, linked to specific symptom patterns. Second, the enteric nervous system has rapidly evolved as a major target for pharmacotherapy of functional gastrointestinal disorders. Pharmacological treatment of gastrointestinal motility disorders is intended to stimulate or inhibit motility. Established sites of action of motility drugs are gastrointestinal smooth muscle, the enteric nervous system, autonomic ganglia and the central nervous system. Compared to agents that act directly at the gastrointestinal smooth muscle (cholinomimetics, nitrates, L-type calcium channel blockers...), stimulation or inhibition of contractile activity through receptors on enteric neuronal circuitry offers the potential of achieving a higher regional and motor response-specificity.

Functional dyspepsia is a clinical syndrome defined by chronic or recurrent upper abdominal symptoms without identifiable cause by conventional diagnostic means. The symptom complex is often related to feeding and includes epigastric pain, fullness, bloating, early satiety, belching, nausea and vomiting [1]. Dyspepsia accounts for 10-20% of general practitioners consultations and about 20-30% of gastroenterological consultations are constituted by patients with functional dyspepsia, indicating that it is a clinical problem of considerable magnitude with obvious implications for the consumption of medical care. Recent studies have established that functional dyspepsia is a heterogeneous disorder, where different pathophysiological disturbances underlie different symptom profiles. Dyspeptic patients with delayed gastric emptying are more likely to suffer from postprandial fullness, nausea and vomiting [4, 5]. Accommodation of the stomach to a meal consists of a relaxation of the proximal stomach, providing the meal with a reservoir and enabling a volume increase without a rise in pressure. Recent studies have established that a subset of dyspeptic patients have impaired accommodation, and this is associated with symptoms of early satiety and weight loss [6]. *Helicobacter pylori* infection in dyspeptic patients is not associated with a specific symptom profile [7]. Finally, patients with hypersensitivity to gastric distension are more likely to suffer from epigastric pain and belching [8].

The idea that functional dyspepsia is a heterogeneous disorder is also reflected in the Rome II criteria, which propose to subdivide functional dyspepsia into ulcer-like dyspepsia (pain is the dominant symptom), motility-like dyspepsia (discomfort type symptoms are the dominant symptom) and unspecified dyspepsia (none of the previous) [1]. However, when applying the Rome II subdivision to 105 consecutive functional dyspepsia patients, we were unable to demonstrate a correlation between the Rome II subdivision, pathophysiological mechanisms, symptom pattern and symptom severity. It seems therefore that a pathophysiology-based approach yields a better subdivision of functional dyspepsia.

Prokinetic drugs, such as cisapride, motilin and erythromycin, stimulate gastrointestinal motility at least in part through the release of acetylcholine from intrinsic cholinergic neurons [9, 10]. In patients with delayed emptying, gastroprokinetic drugs should improve symptoms of postprandial fullness, nausea and vomiting. Studies available so far fail to convincly prove this hypothesis [11, 12]. In patients with impaired accommodation during and after the ingestion of a meal, restoring gastric accommodation is likely to improve symptoms of early satiety. The 5-HT$_4$ receptor agonist cisapride is often used in the treatment of functional dyspepsia. In healthy subjects, we observed that pretreatment with cisapride significantly enhanced the accommodation to a meal [13]. Acute studies with the anti-migraine drug sumatriptan and a therapeutic trial with the anxiolytic drug buspirone established the therapeutic potential of fundus-relaxing 5-HT$_1$ receptor agonists [6, 14]. These agents seem to enhance the release of nitric oxide from intrinsic inhibitory motor neurons [15, 16]. In healthy subjects, pretreatment with the selective serotonin reuptake inhibitor paroxetine is able to strongly enhance the meal-induced relaxation of the proximal stomach [17], but therapeutic trials in functional dyspepsia are still lacking. The treatment of hypersensitivity to gastric distension is more problematic. Recent studies provide evidence that sensitivity to gastric distension is mediated through the activation of in series ("tension") mechanoreceptors in the gastric wall [18]. Tension receptors are inactivated during gastric relaxation, which offers a potential therapeutic approach [19]. Preliminary evidence suggests that fundus-relaxing drugs might improve hypersensitivity to gastric distension and meal-related symptoms in functional dyspepsia [20].

The irritable bowel syndrome (IBS) is probably the most commonly encountered disorder by gastroenterologists in the industrialized world. It is characterized by altered bowel habits, usually with abdominal pain, in the absence of organic disease [2]. Symptoms suggestive of IBS are occur very frequently in the community, but the majority of individuals with IBS symptoms do not consult a doctor. No diagnostic markers for IBS exist, so the diagnosis rests on the recognition of characteristic symptom patterns and the exclusion of organic disease. IBS is characterized by a symptom cluster which includes abdominal pain, often relieved by defecation, distention of the abdomen, a disordered bowel habit, a frequent feeling of incomplete evacuation, mucus in the stool, looser stools with pain onset, and more frequent stools with pain onset. In addition, a number of noncolonic features have also been recognized, including nausea, vomiting, early satiety, nocturia, frequency and urgency of micturition, incomplete bladder emptying and tiredness.

A number of medications have been proposed for the treatment of IBS. However, until recently, the therapeutic effects in the IBS population as a whole were disappointing. Recent developments have focused on alterations in colonic transit to achieve symptomatic benefit in subgroups of IBS patients. Serotonin$_3$ (5-HT$_3$) receptor antagonists inhibit colonic motor activity in man *via* a neural pathway [21]. Recently, the efficacy of alosetron, a 5-HT$_3$ receptor in alleviating symptoms in female IBS patients has been demonstrated [22]. Similarly, 5-HT$_4$ receptor agonists, like tegaserod or prucalopride, enhance colonic transit through the induction of mass movements [23, 24], and preliminary data suggest that these agents may be useful in the treatment of constipation-predominant IBS [25].

Future evolutions in functional bowel disorders are likely to provide simpler tests to assess underlying pathophysiology. Recently developed less invasive techniques, such as gastric emptying breath tests or a caloric satiety test, may facilitate pathophysiological studies in dyspeptic patients [6, 26]. In addition, a wider range of more selectively acting motility modifying drugs will become available.

The selection of a drug therapy with optimal specificity requires a precise knowledge of the circuitry and the receptors that are involved in any given motor phenomenon in man. Unfortunately, our knowledge of the enteric nervous system in man is extremely limited, and most of the information we have available is by extrapolating from animal studies. Studies aimed at mapping enteric neuronal circuitry in man are badly needed. Such studies will be hampered by the limited availability of human tissue for physiological and pharmacological studies and the use fact that techniques used to study the enteric nervous system in small animals are not easily applicable to the human species. Innovative techniques using optical imaging of neuronal activity may have important advantages with that respect [27, 28].

References

1. Talley NJ, Stanghellini V, Heading RC, Koch KL, Malagelada JR, Tytgat GJN. Functional gastroduodenal disorders. *Gut* 1999; 45 (Suppl. II): 37-42.
2. Thompson WG, Longstreth GF, Drossman DA, Heaton KW, Irvine EJ, Muller-Lissner SA. Functional bowel disorders and functional abdominal pain. *Gut* 1999; 45 (Suppl. II): 43-7.

3. Quigley EM. Symptoms and gastric function in dyspepsia-goodbye to gastroparesis? *Neurogastroenterol Motil* 1996; 8: 273-5.
4. Stanghellini V, Tosetti C, Paternico A, Barbara G, Morselli-Labate AM, Monetti N, Mrengo M, Corinaldesi R. Risk indicators of delayed gastric emptying of solids in patients with functional dyspepsia. *Gastroenterology* 1996; 110: 1036-42.
5. Tack J, Caenepeel P, Geypens B, Janssens J. Symptom pattern and gastric emptying rate assessed by the octanoic acid breath test in functional dyspepsia. Submitted for publication.
6. Tack J, Piessevaux H, Coulie B, Caenepeel P, Janssens J. Role of impaired gastric accommodation to a meal in functional dyspepsia. *Gastroenterology* 1998; 115: 1346-52.
7. Tack J, Caenepeel P, Janssens J. Helicobacter pylori, symptom severity and pathophysiological mechanisms in functional dyspepsia. Submitted for publication.
8. Tack J, Caenepeel P, Fischler B, Janssens J. Symptoms associated with hypersensitivity to gastric distension in functional dyspepsia. Submitted for publication.
9. Tonini M, Galligan JJ, North RA. Effects of cisapride on cholinergic neurotransmission and propulsive motility in the guinea-pig ileum. *Gastroenterology* 1989; 96: 1257-64.
10. Tack J. Motilin and the enteric nervous system in the control of interdigestive and postprandial gastric motility. *Acta Gastroenterol Belg* 1995; 1: 21-30.
11. Talley NJ, Verlinden M, Snape W, Becker JA, Ducrotte P, Dettmer A, Brinkhoff H, Eaker E, Ohning G, Miner PB, Mathias JR, Mack RJ. Lack of anti-dyspeptic effects of the macrolide gastrokinetic agent, ABT-229, in functional dyspepsia and idiopathic gastroparesis. *Gastroenteroloy* 2000; 118: A847 (abstract).
12. Sturm A, Holtmann G, Goebell H, Gerken G. Prokinetics in patients with gastroparesis: a systematic analysis. *Digestion* 1999; 60: 422-7.
13. Tack J, Broeckaert D, Coulie B, Janssens J. Influence of cisapride on gastric tone and on the perception of gastric distension. *Aliment Pharmacol Ther* 1998; 12: 761-6.
14. Tack J, Piessevaux H, Coulie B, Caenepeel P, Janssens J. A placebo-controlled trial of buspirone, a fundus-relaxing drug, in functional dyspepsia. Submitted for publication.
15. Coulie B, Tack J, Sifrim D, Andrioli A, Janssens J. Role of nitric oxide in fasting gastric fundus tone and in 5-hydroxytryptamine-1 receptor-mediated relaxation of the gastric fundus. *Am J Physiol* 1999; 276: G373-7.
16. Tack J, Demedts I, Vos R, Meulemans A, Schuurkes J, Janssens J. Role of nitric oxide in the accommodation reflex, in meal-induced satiety and in the treatment of impaired accommodation in man. *Gastroenterology* 2000; 118: A388 (abstract).
17. Tack J, Broeckaert D, Coulie B, Janssens J. Involvement of 5-hydroxytryptamine in the gastric accommodation reflex in man. Submitted for publication.
18. Distrutti E, Azpiroz F, Soldevilla A, Malagelada JR. Gastric wall tension determines perception of gastric distention. *Gastroenterology* 1999; 116: 1035-42.
19. Tack J, Sifrim D. A little rest and relaxation. *Gut* 2000, in press.
20. Tack J, Piessevaux H, Coulie B, Janssens J. Influence of a fundus-relaxing drug on meal-related symptoms in dyspeptic patients with hypersensitivity to gastric distension. Submitted for publication.
21. Talley NJ, Phillips SF, Haddad A, Miller LJ, Twomey C, Zinsmeister AR, MacCarty RL, Ciocola A. GR 38032F (ondansetron), a selective 5-HT3 receptor antagonist, slows colonic transit in healthy man. *Dig Dis Sci* 1990; 35: 477-80.
22. Camilleri M, Northcutt AR, Kong S, Dukes GE, McSorley D, Mangel AW. Efficacy and safety of alosetron in women with irritable bowel syndrome: a randomised, placebo-controlled trial. *Lancet* 2000; 355 (9209): 1035-40.
23. Poen AC, Felt-Bersma RJ, Van Dongen A, Meuwissen SG. Effect of prucalopride, a new enterokinetic agent, on gastrointestinal transit and anorectal function in healthy volunteers. *Aliment Pharmacol Ther* 1999; 13: 1493-7.
24. Scott LJ, Perry CM. Tegaserod. *Drugs* 1999; 58: 491-6.

25. Prather CM, Camilleri M, Zinsmeister AR, McKinzie S, Thomforde G. Tegaserod accelerates orocecal transit in patients with constipation-predominant irritable bowel syndrome. *Gastroenterology* 2000; 118: 463-8.
26. Ghoos YF, Maes BD, Geypens BJ, Hiele MI, Rutgeerts PJ, Vantrappen G. Measurement of gastric emptying rate of solids by means of a carbon labeled octanoic acid breath test. *Gastroenterology* 1993; 104: 1640-7.
27. Neunlist M, Peters S, Schemann M. Multisite optical recording of excitability in the enteric nervous system. *Neurogastroenterol Motil* 1999; 11 (5): 393-402.
28. Vanden Berghe P, Tack J, Coulie B, Andrioli A, Bellon E, Suetens P, Janssens J. Synaptic transmission induces transient calcium concentration changes in cultured myenteric neurons. *Neurogastroenterol Motility* 2000, in press.

Gastrointestinal-safe anti-inflammatory therapy: is it possible?

Carmelo Scarpignato[1,2], Iva Pelosini[1]

[1] Laboratory of Clinical Pharmacology, Department of Internal Medicine, School of Medicine & Dentistry, University of Parma, Italy
[2] Department of Gastroenterology & Hepatology, Faculty of Medicine, University of Nantes, France

The mechanisms involved in the pathogenesis of NSAID-induced gastro-duodenal damage have evolved from the original concept that it resulted from direct topical injury. It is now well established that, in addition to epithelial injury (to which both PG-dependent and PG-independent mechanisms contribute) also a microvascular injury takes place in NSAID-induced gastro-duodenal damage. Each of these mechanisms represents a potential site of pharmacological strategies for prevention.

Since PGs are well established modulators of inflammatory response, it is evident that **NSAIDs induce damage to GI tract *via* a mechanism identical to that by which they exert their anti-inflammatory action.** In this context, it is very difficult to imagine an effective NSAID completely devoid of GI side effects. It should be remembered indeed that any manipulation which alters the ability of an NSAID to inhibit COX activity, and therefore its gastro-duodenal toxicity, will also interfere with the drug's ability to produce its desirable (*i.e.* anti-inflammatory, antipyretic and analgesic) effects.

Although co-therapy with misoprostol or PPIs is effective in preventing NSAID-induced gastroduodenal damage, a more appealing approach would be to develop drugs that are devoid of or have reduced GI toxicity. Currently, selective inhibitors of the inducible cyclo-oxygenase (COX) enzyme offer the best chance for providing patients with an effective and safe anti-inflammatory therapy. Additional compounds that are being developed include nitric oxide-releasing NSAIDs (NO-NSAIDs), dual inhibitors of both cyclo-oxygenase and 5-lypoxygenase as well as NSAIDs which are chemically associated with zwitterionic phospholipids. Finally, although previous attempts have been disappointing, new improved formulations of conventional NSAIDs might have some chance of displaying a reduced topical irritancy.

Highly selective COX-2 inhibitors

Already in 1972, the existence of multiple forms of the enzyme primarily responsible for prostaglandin synthesis was suggested. Flower and Vane observed that while standard NSAIDs inhibited PG synthesis in the brain and peripheral tissues, acetaminophen only exerted inhibitory activity in the brain. In the recent years, the use of molecular biology techniques has allowed the recognition that there are at least two isoforms of COX, the COX-1 and COX-2 isoenzymes, showing about 60% amino acid identity. The COX-1 enzyme is constitutively expressed in most cell types whereas COX-2 is rapidly inducible by lipopolysaccharide (LPS) in monocytes and by interleukin-1 (IL-1) in fibroblasts. Inflammatory tissues, such as synovia of patients with rheumatoid arthritis, express COX-2 message and have COX 2 protein. Moreover, the levels of this enzyme have been shown to be up-regulated at sites of inflammation. COX-2 would appear to fulfil the role of producer of the inflammatory PGs involved in the acute inflammatory response while COX-1 produces the PGs needed for the regulation of important physiological processes as, for instance, maintenance of gastroduodenal mucosal integrity and renal blood flow *(figure 1)*. Thus, it is suppression of COX-1 activity by NSAIDs that is believed to be a crucial factor in the pathogenesis of NSAID-injury. On theoretical grounds, selective COX-2 inhibitors would suppress PG synthesis at sites of inflammation but would spare constitutive PG synthesis in the different tissues, including the GI tract, and therefore would not damage GI mucosa.

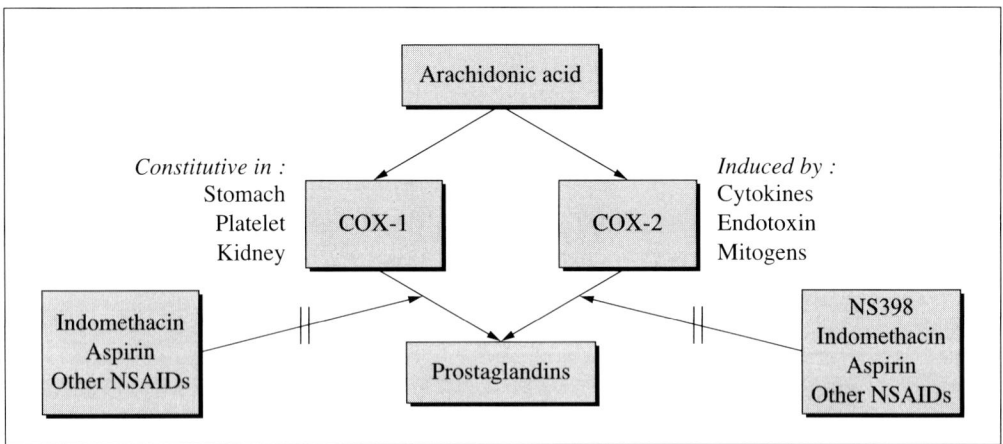

Figure 1. Cyclooxygenase isoforms in mammalian tissues.

After the discovery of COX isoenzymes, new and established NSAIDs were assessed with respect to their relative COX-1/COX-2 selectivities. The basic technique involves comparing IC_{50s} (*i.e.* concentrations need to inhibit by 50% PG production) for COX-1 and COX-2 mediated PGE_2 production in various systems. A COX-2/COX-1 ratio is thus arrived at such that a low ratio implies that the compound is a relatively specific COX-2 inhibitor. Most inhibitors (flurbiprofen, ibuprofen, meclofenamic acid, and docosahexaenoic acid) affect both isoenzymes with near equal potency whereas piroxicam, indomethacin, and sulindac sulfide are more potent COX-1 inhibitors. Very few currently available

NSAIDs (nabumetone, meloxicam, etodolac and nimesulide) show a certain degree of selectivity towards COX-2.

The relative safety of different NSAIDs has been examined in various studies ranging from small-scale volunteer studies of new NSAIDs to large scale epidemiological research. If the relative safety from epidemiological studies is compared with the COX-2/COX-1 ratios of the NSAIDs studied, certain trends do emerge *(figure 2)*. Analysis of the available data indicates the NSAIDs at the safer end of the spectrum appear to be **preferential** COX-2 inhibitors, the term **selective** being reserved to the new compounds (like celecoxib and rofecoxib) whose selectivity ratio is greater than 100 fold for the COX-2 isoenzyme. It must be emphasized, however, that the magnitude of selectivity required from maximum anti-inflammatory efficacy and minimal GI toxicity is presently unknown, being the plasmatic drug levels achieved *in vivo* after administration of therapeutic doses an important co-factor. Furthermore, the diverse systems used to measure COX-1 and COX-2 activities have led to confusing data, the different experimental models yielding a different rank order of COX ratios for different NSAIDs. For instance, the active metabolite of nabumetone, 6-methoxy-2-naphthyl acetic acid (6-NMA), was reported to be a selective inhibitor of murine COX-2, but appears to be less active against human COX-2. Nabumetone, as other currently available preferential COX-2 inhibitors (meloxicam, etodolac and nimesulide, are aggressively marketed as safer NSAIDs but they all are still endowed with a certain degree of GI toxicity.

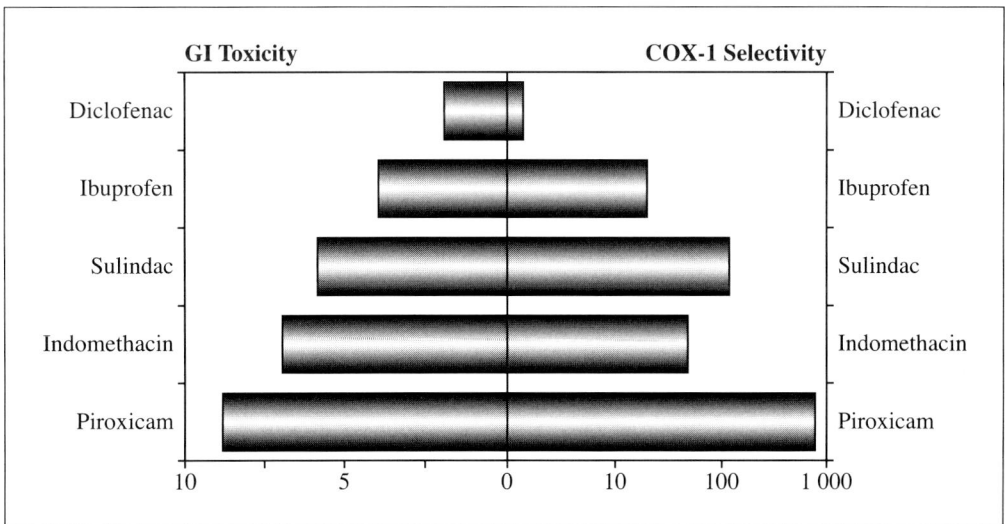

Figure 2. Comparison of gastric damage and COX selectivity of non-steroidal anti-inflammatory drugs (NSAIDs). The left side represents the ranking of drugs according to relative risks of major gastrointestinal complications from a meta-analysis of multi-centre, controlled epidemiological studies. Values for anti-inflammatory doses of NSAIDs are shown. The right side represents log COX-2/COX-1 activity ratios in intact cells (IC_{50} values; μmol/l) for some NSAIDs (from Vane and Botting, 1996).

Two highly selective COX-2 inhibitors [celecoxib (SC 58635) or rofecoxib (MK-966)], which have been shown to spare GI mucosa in experimental animals, have entered clinical trials and are now on the market in USA and some European countries. Single doses of celecoxib (100 or 400 mg) or rofecoxib (50 mg) were superior to placebo and as effective as aspirin or conventional NSAIDs (ibuprofen or naproxen) for pain relief following dental extraction. Phase 2 studies in osteoarthritis (OA) have investigated for celecoxib and rofecoxib dose ranges of 25-200 mg bid and 12.5-25 mg per day, respectively while for the first compound a dose range of 40-400 mg bid was selected for treatment of rheumatoid arthritis. Phase III studies in the above indications have shown that 100-200 mg bid of celecoxib and 12.5-25 mg *per* day of rofecoxib have equivalent efficacy to naproxen 500 mg or diclofenac 75 mg, both twice daily or ibuprofen 800 mg three times a day. Compared with placebo, both celecoxib and rofecoxib improved the quality of life in the physical and mental domains of the SF36 questionnaire.

There are no published data on the effect of celecoxib on prostaglandin synthesis in human gastric mucosa while rofecoxib proved to be unable to affect gastric mucosal PG synthesis or serum TXB2. However, celecoxib did not affect platelet aggregation and bleeding time in healthy volunteers and an acute endoscopic study showed that levels of gastric mucosal injury with celecoxib 100 or 200 mg twice daily for 7 days were similar to those with placebo and significantly lower than those observed with naproxen 500 mg twice a day. Large studies performed in OA and RA patients treated over 3 or 6 months have shown an ulcer incidence that is similar to that with placebo, not dose-related (at least in the range 200-800 mg and significantly lower than that observed with naproxen and diclofenac. Similarly, in doses of 250 mg per day (10-20 times the likely recommended clinical dose), rofecoxib has been well-tolerated, retained COX-1/COX-2 selectivity, with no effect on bleeding time, and caused levels of gastric mucosal injury that were similar to placebo and less than with ibuprofen 2.4 g or aspirin 2.6 g over 7 days. This dose did not significantly increase excretion of ^{51}Cr-labelled red cells over 28 days compared with placebo, while ibuprofen 2.4 g had such an effect. At doses 2-4 times those effective for osteoarthritis, rofecoxib caused significantly less gastroduodenal ulceration than ibuprofen (2.4 g daily), with ulcer rates comparable to placebo. Last but not least, there was no effect on small-intestine permeability over 7 days, by contrast with the significant increases seen with indomethacin 150 mg. However, the incidence of gastric ulceration in patients on concomitant steroids and patients with a recent history of upper GI bleeding from gastric or duodenal ulcerations has not been studied with the newer agents. Patients on low dose aspirin for prevention of cerebrovascular events, and treated with celecoxib, did show an increased incidence of gastric ulcerations when compared with patients only treated with celecoxib. The incidence of significant upper GI bleeding for several thousand patients treated for over six months with celecoxib has been very low, and statistically insignificant, but these patients have been followed for less than two years in most instances. In any case, both drugs carry – at the present time – the normal NSAID warnings about GI effects, although statements about a better tolerability are included in the product labellings. Only post-marketing surveillance data will allow to confirm or withdraw these warnings.

The most common GI side effect associated with celecoxib and rofecoxib in clinical trials has been the development of mild dyspepsia, whose incidence was not however different from that observed in placebo-treated patients. As expected, there was no correlation between dyspeptic symptoms and the incidence of endoscopically observed gastric ulceration or significant blood loss.

While the pursuit of a highly selective COX-2 inhibitors seems a rational approach to developing an NSAID without GI toxicity (both Monsanto Searle and MSD have already described "second-generation" COX-2 inhibitors and several other Drug Companies are developing new compounds), the emerging role of PGs as modulators of mucosal defence in situations where the mucosa is inflamed raises several points that deserve considerations. First, it is possible that prostanoids produced *via* COX-1 contribute to inflammation, pain and fever. There is evidence that COX-1 is up-regulated at sites of inflammation. Selective COX-2 inhibitors would not affect PG synthesis from this enzyme and, therefore, would not be able to counterbalance COX-1 mediated responses. On the other hand, COX-2 might generate endogenous prostanoids that are biologically important. Mice in which the gene for COX-2 has been disrupted have defects in renal function and regulation of bone resorption, and female mice have impaired reproductive physiology. It is also possible that prostanoids derived from COX-2 exert immunomodulatory or cytoprotective effects in situations in which the mucosa is inflamed, such as would be the case in *Helicobacter pylori* associated gastritis or ulcerative colitis. It is well known that NSAIDs can retard, while PGs accelerate ulcer healing. Since existing NSAIDs are effective inhibitors of both COX-1 and COX-2 isoenzymes, it is possible that the retarding effect of NSAIDs on ulcer healing is related to their inhibitory effect on COX-2. In this connection, recent evidence suggests that a COX-2 inhibitor delays ulcer healing significantly less than a predominant COX-1 inhibitor. Since nonselective NSAIDs inhibit COX-2 to varying degrees, the critical factor in determining the inhibitor effect on ulcer healing may be the ratio of isoenzyme inhibition. It has been suggested that an increase in mucosal COX-2 expression may be necessary for the normal healing of gastroduodenal ulcers end experimental studies have shown that COX-2 inhibitors retard ulcer healing. Preliminary data would suggest that this is not the case in humans. Furthermore, COX-2 protein is more prominent than COX-1 in the mucosa of patients with gastric ulcers, representing most likely the major source of PGs in that condition.

McAdam *et al.* recently reported that celecoxib and ibuprofen suppressed the urinary excretion of prostacyclin in healthy subjects, whereas thromboxane activity related to COX-1 was suppressed only by ibuprofen. This effect of COX-2 inhibition has been confirmed with rofecoxib in healthy older adults by the same group of investigators. The authors speculated that long-term therapy with these agents might increase the rate of thrombotic events in patients who were at increased risk for cardiovascular disease, although no data were collected on such events.

As stated by Hawkey, celecoxib and rofecoxib are likely to have a major impact on prescribing in inflammation and analgesia and look set to become the first cyclo-oxygenase inhibitors convincingly to break the prostaglandin-dependent link between efficacy and gastrotoxicity in human beings. However, careful post-marketing surveillance will be important to determine their ultimate benefit and safety profile.

Towards a GI safer NSAID: a look to the future

NO-NSAIDs

NO is now recognized as a critical mediator of GI mucosal defence, exerting many of the same actions as PGs in the GI tract. For instance, PGS and NO are both capable of modulating mucosal blood flow, mucus release, and repair of mucosal injury. Both mediators are also capable of inhibiting neutrophil adherence and activation and mast cell degranulation. In experimental models of gastric injury, NO is capable of exerting cytoprotective effects similar to those observed with PGs. There also appears to be some cooperation between the NO- and PG-mediated components of mucosal defence in that suppression of one arm can lead to an apparently compensatory elevation of the other. Further evidence of the cooperative interactions between NO and PGs in modulating mucosal defence is the evidence that these mediators can regulate the activity of the enzymes responsible for the synthesis of one another.

Because the ulcerogenic effects of NSAIDs are – at least partially – attributable to disturbances in gastric blood flow and reduction of NO synthesis seems to be a pathophysiological mechanism of GI injury by NSAID derivatives which include a NO-releasing moiety (similar to that found in organic nitrates) have been developed in an attempt to develop NSAIDs which do not cause gastric injury. In this connection, Wallace *et al.* reported that nitroxybutylester derivatives of two widely used NSAIDs (namely flurbiprofen and ketoprofen) cause significant less gastric mucosal injury than the parent compounds, despite producing a comparable suppression of PG synthesis and a recent investigation demonstrated that these compounds also spare duodenal mucosa. Moreover, experimental studies have suggested that NO donors, including NO-NSAIDs, can accelerate the healing of preexisting gastric ulcers in a rat model. In a recent seven-day clinical trial, a flurbiprofen-nitric oxide formulation was found to cause fewer gastric erosions than the parent drug, with the same inhibitory effects on gastric mucosal prostaglandin synthesis and serum thromboxane levels. In addition, nitro-aspirin, like aspirin, inhibits platelet aggregation, but it does not suppress cyclooxygenase activity or cause gastric mucosal injury.

Why do NO-NSAIDs not cause gastric damage? As mentioned above, reduced gastric mucosal blood flow after NSAID administration is well documented and may predispose the mucosa to injury induced by topical irritants or endogenous secretions. When NO-NSAIDs are administered, however, gastric mucosal blood flow is maintained at pretreatment levels. Although standard NSAIDs induce neutrophil adherence to the vascular endothelium *(see above)* NO-NSAIDs do not. Both these deleterious effects of NSAIDs could have been counterbalanced by the slow release of NO from NO-NSAIDs. Since NO-donors are able to stimulate mucus secretion and scavenge oxygen-derived free radicals whose generation accounts for mucosal damage, an additional action of released NO at that levels could be envisaged *(figure 3)*. Finally, a very recent investigation showed that NO-aspirin inhibits caspase activity through cGMP-dependent and independent pathways, thus interfering with the apoptotic process.

Dual inhibitors of COX and LO

Compounds with tissue-selective effects on COX (*i.e.* with relatively weak effects on the gastric mucosa and more potent effects at sites of inflammation) may represent a class of NSAIDs without detrimental effects on the stomach and the duodenum. Sodium salicylate, acetaminophen and the recent developed drugs, tepoxalin and ML 3000 belong to this class of drugs. Both these last compounds are also dual inhibitors of COX and 5-LO and they are often referred to as dual-acting anti-inflammatory drugs (DAAIDs). Since LTs

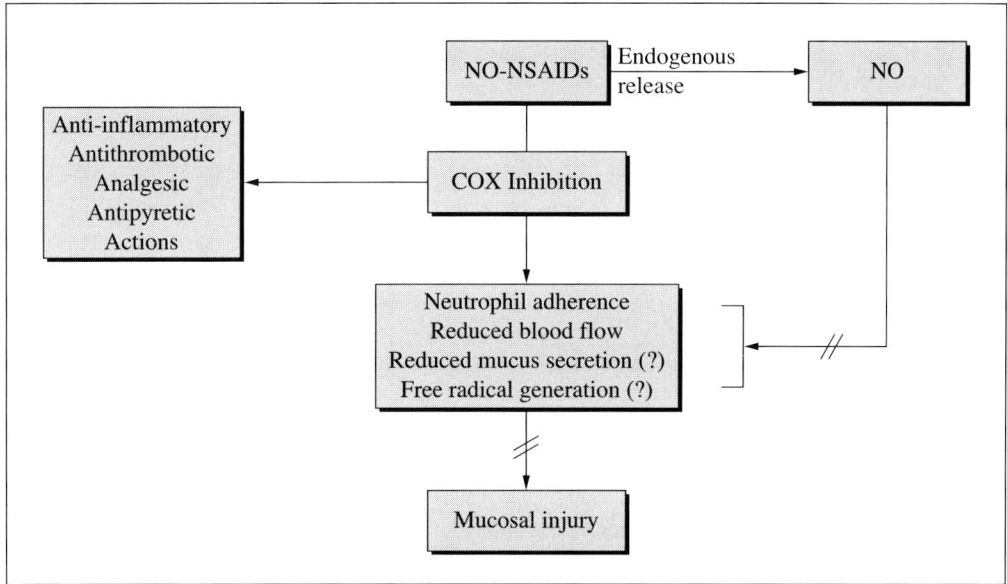

Figure 3. Possible mechanisms underlying the GI safety of NO-NSAIDs (from Wallace, 1997).

are important in the genesis of mucosal damage and LO inhibitors have been shown to reduce the severity of NSAID-induced injury, it is possible that the additional ability of tepoxalin and ML3000 to inhibit 5-LO accounts for their lack of GI side effects. Preliminary studies in healthy volunteers have shown that short-term (4 weeks) administration of ML3000 (either 200 mg or 400 mg bid) spares both gastric and duodenal mucosae. The drug, which is under active development, is now entering phase III clinical trials.

Zwitterionic NSAIDs

It is now well established that mucus layer not only coats the underlying epithelium but also protects it from the cytotoxic effects of the luminal acid. Goddard *et al.* demonstrated about 10 years ago that gastric mucosal hydrophobicity is rapidly attenuated after the mucosa being exposed to acidified ASA and salicylic acid. It was recently shown that certain NSAIDs have a remarkable ability to rapidly complex – in a pH-dependent manner – zwitterionic phospholipids, like for instance phosphatidylcholine, that precipitates out of solution. This chemical association between NSAIDs and gastric surface phospholipids may explain the decline of mucosal hydrophobicity observed after exposure of the gastric mucosa to acidic derivatives.

Based on these observations, Lichtenberger *et al.* proposed that preassociating NSAIDs with zwitterionic phospholipids before their administration should reduce the ability of the NSAIDs to associate with phospholipids in the mucus gel and, therefore, should reduce their ulcerogenicity. They tested this hypothesis by preassociating aspirin and other NSAIDs with dipalmitoylphosphatidylcholine (DPPC). In contrast to the decrease in the hydrophobicity of the gastric mucosal surface (increased contact angle) observed with regular aspirin, the aspirin-DPPC complex had no effect. Moreover, although standard aspirin caused significant GI bleeding, leading to a decrease in hematocrit, aspirin-DPPC did not change this parameter. Not only the preassociation of aspirin with DPPC did not interfere with the effectiveness of aspirin to reduce fever or inflammation, it actually enhanced its effectiveness. A recent, double-blind, short-term study did show that – although aspirin and aspirin-DPPC reduce antral PG content to the same extent – the number of gastric erosions seen with the aspirin-DPPC formulation was significantly less compared with aspirin alone.

Pure enantiomers of chiral NSAIDs

Most chiral NSAIDs are currently administered as racemates containing equal portions of the R- and S-effective enantiomers. It has been demonstrated that the S-enantiomer consistently shows much greater activity in blocking prostaglandin synthesis than the R-enantiomer. Therefore, some companies began making pure S-enantiomers to get rid of the "contaminant" R-enantiomer. However, when the activity of the R-enantiomer of flurbiprofen was examined, it was found to exert analgesic NSAID-effects comparable to the S-enantiomer but because it was a much weaker inhibitor of prostaglandin synthesis, it was proposed to be less ulcerogenic. This led some pharmaceutical companies to develop R-enantiomers of chiral NSAIDs as analgesics. One of such compound (*i.e.* dexketoprofen trometamol) has been marketed in some European countries and found to be well tolerated, with a reported incidence of adverse events similar to that of placebo. It should be noted, however, that some studies have shown that R-enantiomers of flurbiprofen, etodolac, ketoprofen, and ibuprofen are not without adverse effects in the GI tract and are capable of increasing small intestinal permeability in a comparable manner to the S-enantiomer or the racemic preparation. There is also some concern regarding inversion from the R- to the S-enantiomer *in vivo*. Of course, because of their weak activity as COX inhibitors, the R-enantiomers are not very potent anti-inflammatory drugs.

New NSAID formulations

Topical irritancy is one of the mechanisms by which NSAIDs damage gastroduodenal mucosa and represents therefore a target for pharmacological strategies for prevention. It has been attempted with limited success to decrease contact time of NSAIDs with the gastric mucosa through the use of enteric-coated preparation. In the early 80s multiparticulate microsphere dosage forms have been described, which caused a reduced gastric irritation when compared with standard formulations. A more recent approach has been to decrease drug crystal particle size so that there is no longer a large enough crystal lodged against the mucosa to produce a local high concentration and consequent irritation. Reducing drug particle size from 20-30 μm to 270 nm results in a better tolerability and increased absorption. This **NanoCrystal formulation** is now entering clinical trials.

An enhanced pharmacological action and adverse effect reduction can also be obtained relying on specific drug delivery systems. A recent developed lipo-preparation is made of lecithin-coated lipid fine grains containing soybean oil where the drug has been dissolved. A similar preparation with steroids has previously been found extremely effective since lipid microspheres will accumulate at inflammation sites and be taken up by inflammatory cells. A lipo-preparation of flurbiprofen axetil (lipid soluble ester of flurbiprofen), administered by intravenous route, is now available. It has been used as an effective analgesic (its action being stronger than that of other NSAIDs and comparable to that of pentazocine) for more than 4 years with a remarkably low incidence (1.3%) of GI adverse effects. Since NSAIDs are very useful drugs to manage post-operative pain, development of **lipo-NSAID preparations** of other currently available compounds seems worthwhile.

Conclusions

There is little doubt that the key for preventing NSAID-associated gastroduodenal damage relies in a better understanding of the underlying mechanisms for their GI toxicity. Although in the past some drugs were claimed to spare the GI tract, their promises have been mostly unfulfilled. Nowadays, several approaches to the rational design of GI-sparing NSAIDs have shown promise in experimental studies and clinical data with highly selective COX-2 inhibitors showed that they are effective and safe alternatives to existing NSAIDs in the treatment of inflammatory conditions. Paradoxically, the availability of celecoxib and rofecoxib appears to have stimulated the switch of many NSAIDs from the prescription to OTC status. Since OTC availability of NSAIDS exceeds prescription NSAID use by 7 fold, it is conceivable that the reduced GI toxicity from prescribed medication could be reciprocated by a rising problem of ulcer complications due to self-medication. To prevent this "emerging epidemic" we must always rely on a better prescribing policy for the general population and on prophylactic co-therapy in patients at risk.

Key references

- Donnelly MT, Hawkey CJ. COX-II inhibitors – a new generation of safer NSAIDs? *Aliment Pharmacol Ther* 1997; 11: 227-36.
- Hawkey CJ. COX-2 inhibitors. *Lancet* 1999; 353: 307-14.
- Lancaster C. Effective nonsteroidal anti-inflammatory drugs devoid of gastrointestinal side effects. Do they really exist? *Dig Dis* 1995; 13 (Suppl. 1): 40-7.
- Lipsky PE, Abramson SB, Crofford L, Dubois RN, Simon LS, van de Putte LBA. The classification of cyclooxygenase inhibitors. *J Rheumatol* 1998; 25: 2298-302.
- Masferrer JL, Isakson PC, Seibert K. Cyclooxygenase-2 inhibitors. A new class of anti-inflammatory agents that spare the gastrointestinal tract. *Gastroenterol Clin North Am* 1996; 25: 363-72.
- Scarpignato C. Nonsteroidal anti-inflammatory drugs: how do they damage gastroduodenal mucosa? *Dig Dis* 1995; 13 (Suppl. 1): 9-39.
- Scarpignato C. NSAID-induced gastro-duodenal Damage: From Pathogenesis to Prevention. In: Galmiche JP, ed. *Recent advances in the pathophysiology of gastro-intestinal and liver Diseases*. Paris: John Libbey Eurotext, 1997: 47-84.
- Scarpignato C, Pelosini I. Prevention and treatment of non-steroidal anti-inflammatory drug-induced gastro-duodenal damage: rationale for the use of antisecretory compounds. *Ital J Gastroenterol Hepatol* 1999; 31 (Suppl. 1): S63-S72.
- Scarpignato C, Biarnason I, Bretagne JF, de Pouvourville G, García Rodríquez LA, Goldstein JL, Müller P, Simon B. Working Team Report: Towards a GI safer antiinflammatory therapy. *Gastroenterol Int* 1999; 12: 186-215.

- Vane JR, Botting RM. The history of anti-inflammatory drugs and their mechanism of action. In: Bazan N, Botting J, Vane J, eds. New targets in inflammation: inhibitors of COX-2 or adhesion molecules. Dordrecht : Kluwer Academic Publishers, 1996: 1-12.
- Wallace JL, Del Soldato P, Cirino G: Development of NSAIDs with reduced gastrointestinal and renal toxicity. *Exp Opin Invest Drugs* 1995; 4: 613-9.
- Wallace JL. Nonsteroidal anti-inflammatory drugs and gastroenteropathy: the second hundred years. *Gastroenterology* 1997; 112: 1000-16.

Strategies against *H. pylori* infection

Irène Corthésy-Theulaz[1], André Blum[1], Pierre Michetti[2]

[1] Division of Gastroenterology, Centre Hospitalier Universitaire Vaudois, Lausanne, Switzerland
[2] Division of Gastroenterology, Beth Israel Deaconess Medical Center and Harvard Medical School, Boston, MA, USA

The treatment of *H. pylori* infection has evolved from bismuth-based triple drug regimens to the widely accepted proton pump inhibitor (PPI) or ranitidine bismuth citrate (RBC) single week triple therapies. Current triple therapies are well tolerated and provide consistent high cure rates in clinical trials, but several challenges remain. Cure rates tend to be lower in clinical practice than in clinical trials, antibiotic resistance is increasing in most countries, triple therapy is cumbersome, and re-treatment after eradication failure is difficult. For these reasons, research towards better therapies against *H. pylori* is needed. Several new approaches are possible and currently under investigation.

Antibiotic-based therapies

The first line therapy generally accepted as the standard of care for the treatment of *H. pylori* infection is a triple therapy that includes a PPI or RBC in combination with two antibiotics. The recommended antibiotics include amoxicillin, clarithromycin, and metronidazole. The efficacy of these therapies, however, is compromised by antibiotic resistance, that has been demonstrated to all of these antibiotics [1]. Quadruple therapy is currently the recommended second line therapy. Some experts, however, advocate that quadruple therapy should be used as first line therapy in areas of high resistance rates, to avoid treatment failure, with the added advantage of preventing the development of secondary resistance [2]. Concerning the classical PPI-antibiotic approach, novel therapies are likely to be derived from improved combinations of existing antibiotics and from the use of a few novel antibiotics.

New targets defined by genetics

To date the goal of deriving *Helicobacter*-specific therapies from its genome analysis has not been achieved in clinical practice, but several genes and metabolic pathways of the pathogen are recognized as potential targets for drug development. One example of this is the *ureI* gene. This gene belongs to the urease cluster, encodes for a H^+-gated urea channel and has been shown to be essential for *H. pylori* internal pH homeostasis and for intragastric survival [3]. Other possible targets are the succinyl CoA-transferase and the keto-thiolase of *H. pylori*; these two enzymes belong to an enzymatic pathway that is essential for survival of the bacterium and inhibitors of this family of enzymes are available [4]. Other metabolic pathways of *H. pylori* might be accessible to specific inhibition, but the expenses associated with new drug development may limit these genetically-based approaches.

Vaccines

Prophylactic and therapeutic immunization has been successful in animal models, including in the setting of natural infections such as *H. mustelae* in ferrets and *H. pylori* in rhesus monkeys [5]. Despite the obvious limits in extrapolating these results to humans, the repeated success of anti-*Helicobacter* immunization constitutes a proof of principle of this approach for the treatment of *H. pylori* infection.

Various formulations, delivery systems, and routes of immunization have tested the value of *H. pylori* urease in animals, and four clinical trials have been conducted with urease-based vaccines in humans. These studies suggest that urease is safe and immunogenic in humans, but efficacy data are still lacking [6]. The optimal adjuvant and route of immunization to elicit a protective immune response in the human stomach is not yet defined, but further animal studies and clinical trials addressing these questions are in progress. An interesting approach is to use attenuated live bacteria such as modified *Salmonella typhimurium* strains, to express and deliver *H. pylori* antigens [7]. Potentially toxic adjuvants such as cholera toxin may not be required, but if deemed necessary to modulate the immune response, recombinant adjuvants could be included in the system. Furthermore, using this approach, the number of immunizations needed should be few. All the above advantages should result in lower costs, a crucial aspect of vaccine development. The down side of life vaccines, however, is the release of genetically-modified organisms in the wild, with a risk of recombination among bacteria species. This risk may be increased further if virulence factors are used as vaccine antigens. Two studies have recently modeled the cost-effectiveness of a *H. pylori* vaccine. It appears to be a clear benefit in pursuing vaccine development in the industrialized world. However, in developing countries with the highest prevalence of *H. pylori* and scarce public resources, *H. pylori* vaccination compares unfavorably with vaccination against other infectious diseases that cause higher morbidity and mortality in those areas. Development of cheap multivalent vaccines active against several pathogens may overcome these economic obstacles. In addition, recent evidence suggests that *H. pylori* infection may favor and worsen the outcome of other enteric infections, enhancing the potential health benefits of anti-*Helicobacter* vaccination [8].

Anti-adhesion and mucosal protective agents

The ability of *H. pylori* to adhere to gastric cells *via* several receptors, including Lewis X and Y blood group antigens may be essential for sustained infection and *H. pylori*-induced disease. Prevention of *H. pylori* binding to gastric epithelial cells could thus represent a potential target for therapy. This hypothesis has been tested recently in *H. pylori*-infected rhesus monkeys, using 3'- sialyllactose sodium salt. This oligosaccharide that occurs naturally in human and bovine milk, is recognized by *H. pylori* and inhibits adhesion of the bacterium to human epithelial cells *in vitro*. Administration of this adhesion molecule analog resulted in cure of the infection in a few animals, suggesting that this approach may have merit [9]. Lewis, BabA and AlpAB analogs represent other possible decoy molecules. The exact role of Lewis binding in humans, however, is still controversial.

Probiotics

Probiotics, including nonpathogenic strains of *E. coli, lactobacilli*, and the yeast *Saccharomyces boulardii* have been used for decades to combat infectious diseases but, till recently, their benefit was difficult to confirm in randomized trials. Limited information is available regarding the potential benefit of these compounds in *H. pylori* infection. In one randomized, placebo controlled trial, a whey-based culture supernatant of *L. acidophilus (johnsonii)* strain La1 had a sustained suppressive effect on gastric *H. pylori* infection in humans [10]. More recent data suggest that administration of yogurts prepared with this strain decreases *H. pylori* colonization density and gastric inflammation. As increased density of *H. pylori* on the gastric mucosa is associated with more severe gastritis and increased incidence of peptic ulcers, reduction of the infection density by dietary measures might help to decrease the risk of developing gastroduodenal diseases. The mechanisms by which *lactobacilli* suppress *H. pylori* growth remain unclear, but lactic acid production may contribute to this effect. Further understanding of the mechanisms of action of probiotics may lead to effective therapies. These agents may also be used in the future for the delivery of vaccines or other biologically active molecules that expand our armamentarium against *H. pylori*.

References

1. Dore MP, Leandro G, Realdi G, Sepulveda AR, Graham DY. Effect of pretreatment antibiotic resistance to metronidazole and clarithromycin on outcome of *Helicobacter pylori* therapy: a meta-analytical approach. *Dig Dis Sci* 2000; 45: 68-76.
2. O'Morain C, Montague S. Challenges to therapy in the future. *Helicobacter* 2000: 5: 23-6.
3. Weeks DL, Eskandari S, Scott DR, Sachs G. A H^+-gated urea channel: the link between *Helicobacter pylori* urease and gastric colonization. *Science* 2000: 287: 482-5.
4. Corthésy-Theulaz I, Bergonzelli GB, Henry H, Bachmann D, Schorderet DF, Blum AL, Ornston LN. Cloning and characterization of *Helicobacter pylori* succinyl CoA-transferase, a novel prokaryotic member of the CoA transferase family. *J Biol Chem* 1997: 272; 25659-67.

5. Lee A. Vaccines. *Eur J Gastroenterol Hepatol* 1999; 11 (Suppl 2): S75-9.
6. Michetti P, Kreiss K, Kotloff KL, Porta N, Blanco JL, Bachmann D, Saldinger PF, Corthésy-Theulaz I, Losonsky G, Nichols R, Stolte M, Monath TP, Ackermann S, Blum AL. Oral immunization with recombinant urease and *E. coli* heat-labile enterotoxin adjuvant is safe and immunogenic in *Helicobacter pylori* infected adults. *Gastroenterology* 1999: 116; 804-12.
7. Gomez-Duarte OG, Bumann D, Meyer TF. The attenuated Salmonella vaccine approach for the control of *Helicobacter pylori*-related diseases. *Vaccine* 1999; 17: 1667-73.
8. Stratton KR, Durch JS, Lawrence RS. Vaccines for the 21st century: a tool for decision making. Washington DC, National Academy Press, 2000, in press. http://bob.nap.edu/readingroom/books/vacc21.
9. Mysore JV, Wigginton T, Simon PM, Zopf D, Herman-Ackah LM, Dubois A. Treatment of *Helicobacter pylori* infection in rhesus monkeys using a novel antiadhesion compound. *Gastroenterology* 1999; 117: 1316-25.
10. Michetti P, Dorta G, Brassard D, Verdu E, Tappy L, Herranz M, Vouillamoz D, Schwitzer W, Felley C, Porta N, Rouvet W, Blum AL, Corthésy-Theulaz I. Supernatant of whey-based cultures of *Lactobacillus acidophilus* La 1 as an adjuvant in the therapy of *Helicobacter pylori* infection in humans. *Digestion* 1999; 60: 203-9.

Novel approaches in the treatment of gastrointestinal and liver disease: a look into the future.
Galmiche J.P., ed. John Libbey Eurotext, Paris © 2000, pp. 23-27.

Immunomodulation in inflammatory bowel diseases

Pierre Desreumaux

Laboratoire de Recherche sur les Maladies Inflammatoires Intestinales, CHU Lille, France

Crohn's disease (CD) is a chronic inflammatory bowel disease (IBD) characterized by multiple recurrences, which may be endoscopic or clinical. The primary mechanisms leading to the initiation and perpetuation of the inflammatory processes in CD are poorly known. However, it is widely thought that disease initiation and pathogenesis is multifactorial, involving genetic predisposition, environmental factors including bacterial agents and dysregulation of the intestinal immune system.

Cytokine profile expression during the different stages of Crohn's disease

Control of cytokine balance is one of the major regulatory mechanisms in the immune system. The T helper (Th)-1 and Th-2 cytokine patterns are known to determine the nature of the immune response. The Th-1 cytokine profile is characterized by the synthesis of interleukin-2 (IL-2) and interferon-gamma (IFN-γ) whereas the Th-2-type immune response is associated with the production of IL-4, IL-5, IL-13 and supports the switch to IgE isotypes.

Cytokine studies may further enhance our understanding of CD pathogenesis. Accumulated results from these patients indicated that chronic intestinal lesions are associated with a Th-1 cytokine profile [1, 2]. However, the established intestinal lesions reflect a dynamic process of inflammation and healing that involves distinct cellular and molecular mediators. These multiple gut involvements in CD make it difficult to analyze the early pathological events leading to the inflammatory process. Endoscopic recurrences after radical surgery for CD is one of the best situations for studying the pathogenesis of initial lesions of CD [3]. Using the human model of intestinal recurrences after radical surgery, we have demonstrated that divergent mucosal cytokine patterns evolved during the different stages of CD [4]. Early ileal lesions of CD occurring three months after surgery are characterized by an important mucosal eosinophil infiltration (more than 80% of the inflammatory cell population), which correlates with a Th-2 cytokine profile and particularly with an increase of IL-4 and IgE mRNA and a decrease of IFN-γ mRNA. Using immunohistochemistry, the cellular sources of IL-4 were detected as CD4 T cells (70%), mast cells (20%) and eosinophils (10%) [4]. The recruitment of eosinophils in intestinal tissues at this stage of the disease was also associated with an overproduction of CC chemokines and their receptors such as eotaxin, MCP-4, RANTES and CCR-3. In contrast with early lesions of CD, the cellular infiltrate in the chronic mucosal lesions was composed prominantly by neutrophils and macrophages [4]. The cytokine patterns were also completely different with an upregulation of Th-1 cytokines (IL-2 and IFNγ) and inflammatory mediators such as TNFα, IL-1β, IL-8, GRO, MCP-1, MIP-1 α et β, and ENA78 [4]. Mechanisms involved in the switch from a Th-2 to a Th-1 cytokine pattern are poorly understood but may involve an overproduction of IL-18, IL-12 or its β2 chain receptor [5, 6].

Immunomodulation in inflammatory bowel diseases

Salicylates, corticosteroids and immunosuppressive drugs are the main medical treatments for IBD. These drugs are effective because they act non specifically at various sites of the inflammatory cascade. The better knowledge of the mechanisms involved in intestinal inflammation in animal models of colitis and in patients with IBD has led to the development of new specific therapeutic molecules.

The first of the new drugs to reach the market targets TNFα *(figure 1)*. In IBD, chimeric antibodies directed against TNFα (Infliximab) are effective for treatment of 1) moderately to severely active CD in patients who have an inadequate response to conventional therapy [7] and 2) patients with fistulizing CD [8] *(table I)*. Other strategies to restrain inflammation mediated by TNFα are also generating excitement and clinical trials in CD. New humanized antibodies directed against TNFα (CDP571) [9, 10], immunoglobulin fusion proteins including recombinant human TNFα receptor p75 (Etanercept) or p55 (Lenercept) receptors, and Thalidomide are under investigations in IBD [11, 12].

Few published studies have also shown the efficacy of other anti-inflammatory molecules or specific inhibitors of the inflammatory mediators thought to be involved at least in part in CD. More than 400 patients with CD have received subcutaneously recombinant human IL-10, a mediator involved in the regulation of pro-inflammatory and immunoregulatory cytokines *(table II)* [13]. IL-11, a cytokine with thrombocytopoietic and anti-inflammatory activities having a mucosal protective effects, has been also evaluated in patients with CD *(table II)* [14]. Antibodies (Antegren) directed against α4β7 or antisense oligonucleotides (ISIS 2302) of intercellular adhesion molecule (ICAM)-1, two molecules playing an important role in the trafficking of leukocytes in CD, seem to be efficient in those patients *(table II)* [15, 16].

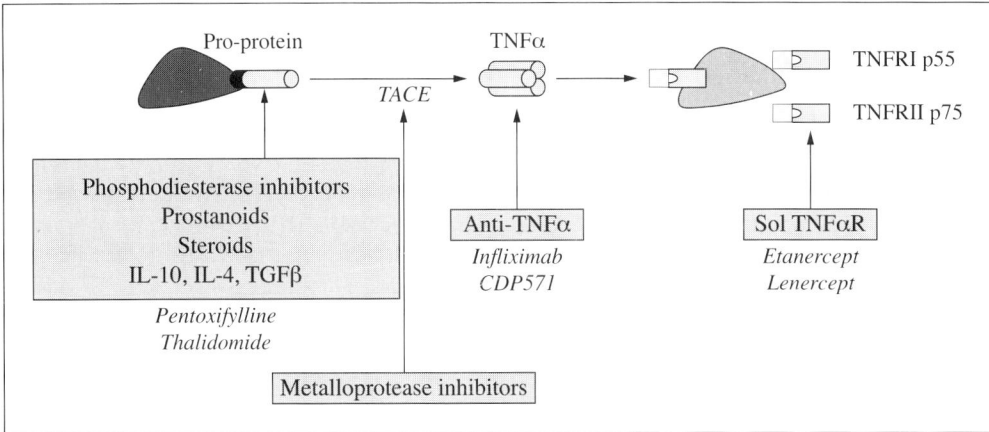

Figure 1. Therapeutic targeting of tumor necrosis factor (TNF)α activity.
TNFα is produced by many cells as a pro-protein which is cleaved by a specific metalloprotease also named TNFα converting enzyme (TACE) to yield a functional TNFα protein. TNFα effects are transmitted via crosslinking of the membrane bound receptor molecules TNF receptor I and II (TNFRI and TNFRII). Anti-TNFα agents can be classified into 4 groups: 1) molecules such as phosphodiesterase inhibitors, prostanoids, corticosteroids, interleukin (IL)-10 and transforming growth factor (TGF)-α which inhibit the production of the pro-protein; 2) inhibitors of the TNFα metalloprotease which affect the processing of the pro-protein; 3) antibodies directed against TNFα and 4) soluble TNF receptors having the ability to bind and inactivate TNFα.

Table I. Efficiency of Infliximab in Crohn's disease (CD)

Moderately-severely active CD	
Recommended administration	2 hours IV injection
Dose	5 mg/kg
Clinical response at 4 and 12 weeks (dCDAI > 70)	81% and 48%
Clinical remission at 4 and 12 weeks (CDAI < 150)	48% and 30%
Fistulizing CD	
Recommended administration	3 IV injections (day 0, W2, W6)
Dose	5 mg/kg
Closure of at least 50% of fistulas at 4 weeks	68%
Closure of all fistulas at 4 weeks	55%
Mean duration of the response	84 days

Table II. Efficiency of new potential drugs in moderately to severely active Crohn's disease (CD)

	Administration	Clinical response Treatment vs placebo	References
IL-10	Subcutaneous	30% vs 10%	[13]
IL-11	Subcutaneous	37% vs 7%	[14]
ISIS	Intravenous	47% vs 20%	[16]
Antegren	Subcutaneous	40% vs 8%	[15]

In animal models with colitis, a lot of molecules are also potentially promising and many clinical trials in patients with CD are in progress. The major source of interest is the used of humanised antibodies directed against IL-12 [17], IL-18 and IFNγ, three key factors involved in the Th-1 cytokine profile. Trials using antisense oligonucleotides of p65, a subunit of NF-κB or anti-oxydant enzyme inhibiting NF-κB (OXIS) are now in a phase II trials in patients with IBD [18]. More recently, different studies have showed that agonists (Thiazolinediones) of a nuclear receptor namely peroxysome proliferator activated receptor (PPAR)-γ protect against colon inflammation in mice [19, 20]. This receptor is mainly expressed in the colon and has anti-inflammatory functions. A trial with PPARγ agonist is now performed in patients with UC.

References

1. Niessner M, Volk BA. Altered Th1/Th2 cytokines profiles in the intestinal mucosa of patients with inflammatory bowel disease as assessed by quantitative reversed transcribed polymerase chain reaction (RT-PCR). *Clin Exp Immunol* 1995; 101: 428-35.
2. Mullin GE, Maycon ZR, Braun-Elwert L, et al. Inflammatory bowel disease mucosal biopsies have specialized lymphokine mRNA profiles. *Inflammatory Bowel Diseases* 1996; 2: 16-26.
3. Rutgeerts P, Geboes K, Vantrappen G, Beyls J, Kerremans R, Hiele M. Predictability of the postoperative course of Crohn's disease. *Gastroenterology* 1990; 99: 956-63.
4. Desreumaux P, Brandt E, Gambiez L, et al. Distinct cytokine patterns in early and chronic ileal lesions of Crohn's disease. *Gastroenterology* 1997; 113: 118-26.
5. Monteleone G, Biancone L, Marasco R, et al. Interleukin 12 is expressed and actively released by Crohn's disease intestinal lamina propria mononuclear cells. *Gastroenterology* 1997; 112: 1169-78.
6. Pizarro TT, Michie MH, Bentz M, et al. IL-18, a novel immunoregulatory cytokine, is up-regulated in Crohn's disease: expression and localization in intestinal mucosal cells. *J Immunol* 1999; 162: 6829-35.
7. Targan SR, Hanauer SB, van Deventer SJH, et al. A short term study of chimeric monoclonal antibody to cA2 to tumour necrosis factor α for Crohn's disease. *N Engl J Med* 1997; 337: 1029-35.
8. Present DH, Rutgeerts P, Targan S, et al. Infliximab for the treatment of fistula in patients with Crohn's disease. *N Engl J Med* 1999; 340: 1398-405.
9. Stack WA, Mann SD, Roy AJ, et al. Randomised controlled trial of CDP571 antibody to tumour necrosis factor-α in Crohn's disease. *Lancet* 1997; 349: 521-4.
10. Feagan BG, Sandborn WJ, Baker JP, et al. A randomized double blind placebo controlled multicenter trial of the engineered human antibody to TNF (CDP571) for steroid sparing and steroid-dependent Crohn's disease. *Gut* 1999; 45: A131.
11. Ehrenpreis ED, Kane SV, Cohen LB, Cohen RD, Hanauer SB. Thalidomide therapy for patients with refractory Crohn's disease: an open – label trial. *Gastroenterology* 1999; 117: 1271-7.
12. Vasiliauskas EA, Kam LY, Abreu-Martin MT, et al. An open-label pilot study of low dose thalidomide in chronically active, steroid-dependent Crohn's disease. *Gastroenterology* 1999; 117: 1278-87.
13. Schreiber S, Fedorak RN, Wild G, et al. Safety and tolerance of rHuIL-10 treatment in patients with mild/moderate active ulcerative colitis. *Gastroenterology* 1998; 114: G4424.
14. Sands BE, Bank S, Sninsky CA, et al. Preliminary evaluation of safety and activity of recombinant human interleukin-11 in patients with active Crohn's disease. *Gastroenterology* 1999; 117: 58-64
15. Gordon FH, Lai CWY, Hamilton MI, et al. Randomised double-blind placebo controlled trial of recombinant humanised antibody to α4 integrin (Antegren™) in active Crohn's disease. *Gastroenterology* 1999; 116: G3152.

16. Yacyshyn BR, Bowen-Yacyshyn MB, Jewel L, *et al.* A placebo controlled trial of ICAM-1 antisense oligonucleotide in the treatment of Crohn's disease. *Gastroenterology* 1998; 114: 1133-42.
17. Fuss I, Marth T, Neurath MF, Pearlstein GR, Jain A, Strober W. Anti-interleukin 12 treatment regulates apoptosis of Th1 T cells in experimental colitis in mice. *Gastroenterology* 1999; 117: 1078-88.
18. Neurath MF, Pettersson S, Meyer zum Buschenfelde KH, Strober W. Local administration of antisense phosphorothioate oligonucleotides to the p65 subunit of NF-kappa B abrogates established experimental colitis in mice. *Nature Med* 1996; 2: 998-1004.
19. Su CG, Wen X, Bailey ST, *et al.* A novel therapy for colitis utilizing PPAR-gamma ligands to inhibit the epithelial inflammatory response. *J Clin Invest* 1999; 104: 383-9.
20. Dubuquoi L, Desreumaux P, Peuchmaur M, Nutten S, Colombel JF, Auwerx J. Preventive and curative effects of PPARγ activators in TNBS colitis through inhibition of TNFα. *Gut* 1999; 45: A34.

Probiotics in inflammatory bowel diseases

Paolo Gionchetti

Department of Internal Medicine and Gastroenterology, University of Bologna, Italy

A body of evidence from clinical and experimental observations indicates a role for intestinal microflora in the pathogenesis of inflammatory bowel diseases (IBD). The distal ileum and the colon are the areas with highest luminal bacterial concentration, and represent the sites of inflammation in IBD. Similarly, pouchitis, a non-specific inflammation of the ileal reservoir, appears to be associated with high bacterial concentrations. Enteric bacteria and their products have been detected within inflamed mucosa in Crohn's disease and recently it has been shown that luminal content, presumably dominated by bacteria, is able to trigger post-operative recurrence of Crohn's disease in the terminal ileum within a few days. Recent studies have shown convincing evidence of a breakdown of tolerance to the normal commensal flora in active IBD, supporting the theory that hyperactivity to ubiquitous antigens from the intestinal microflora is implicated at least in perpetuation of IBD. Suppression of the microflora with antibiotics, faecal stream diversion and bowel rest decrease activity of Crohn's disease, but has less effect in patients with ulcerative colitis. Patients with pouchitis may also be effectively treated with antibiotics. Purified bacterial products can initiate and perpetuate experimental colitis. Finally, it has been noted that the spontaneous colitis that consistently develops in many transgenic and knock-out mutant murine models of colitis, may not occur when these lines are maintained in germ-free conditions.

Earlier in the century, the Russian Nobel-prize Laureate, Elie Metchnikoff first suggested that high numbers of lactobacilli were important in the intestinal flora for health and longevity of humans. In the same period Tissier showed that bifidobacteria were the predominant flora in breast-fed infants, and it was speculated that infant diarrhoea could be treated by giving large doses of bifidobacteria orally.

Probiotics are living organisms, which upon ingestion in certain numbers, exert health benefits beyond inherent basic nutrition. Most of probiotics belong to a large group of bacteria, designated as lactic acid bacteria (lactobacilli and bifidobacteria), that are important components of the human gastrointestinal microflora where they exist as harmless commensals. Probiotic strains must be of human origin, because some health-promoting effects may be species-specific. Other required properties include acid and bile resistance, ability to survive and be metabolically active within the intestinal lumen, where they should not persist long-term. Probiotic strains must also be antagonistic against pathogenic bacteria either by producing antimicrobial substances, or by competitive exclusion or promoting a reduction of luminal colonic pH. Obviously, they must be safe and tested for human use. Different strains of probiotic bacteria have very different and specialised functions. Most of the data we have about probiotics are coming from experimental conditions and a lot of scepticism is diffused among researchers mainly because the mechanisms by which probiotic bacterial strains antagonise pathogenic gastro-intestinal micro-organisms or exert other beneficial effects in the host *in vivo*, have not been fully defined yet.

Very few data are now available on the role of probiotics in experimental and human IBD. Two studies have shown a significant decrease in lactobacilli concentration in colonic biopsies from patients with active ulcerative colitis and also pouchitis is associated with reduced counts of lactobacilli and bifidobacteria. In patients with Crohn's disease it has been reported a decrease of bifidobacteria fecal concentration and oral administration of *Lactobacillus GG* has resulted in an increase in the intestinal IgA immune response.

Exogenous administration of different strains of lactobacilli was shown to prevent the development of acetic acid-induced colitis, methotrexate-induced colitis and of spontaneous colitis in IL-10 deficient mice. In two recent controlled studies, one carried out for 3 months and the other for one year, patients with ulcerative colitis were given oral mesalazine or capsules containing a non-pathogenic strain of *E. coli* (Nissle, 1917) as maintenance treatment. No significant difference in relapse rate was observed between the two treatments. This non-pathogenic strain of *E. coli* was isolated by Alfred Nissle in 1917 from the faeces of a pioneer officer, who, in contrast of his companions, was not affected during an epidemic dysentery infection.

We have recently explored another strategy, using a probiotic preparation (VSL#3) characterised by a high bacterial concentration (300 billions/g of viable lyophilised micro-organisms) and the presence of a mixture of different bacterial species. The rationale for this approach was to try to manipulate the intestinal microflora by influencing its microbial composition through both the high number of bacteria and the possible synergistic action of the different strains. In two studies, using this probiotic preparation, in patients with ulcerative colitis (UC) and pouchitis in remission, a significant increase in ingested probiotic strains was found in stool of these patients together with a significant decrease of stool pH. In the pouchitis study, patients treated with probiotics had a significant better outcome than those who received placebo. This positive effect of VSL#3 was recently confirmed in the prevention of pouchitis onset in patients operated of ileal-pouch anal anastomosis for UC. Patients treated with VSL#3 had a significantly lower incidence of pouchitis compared with those treated with placebo during the first year after ileostomy closure.

With regard to the mechanism of action of VSL#3, we also have found a significant increase in tissue levels of IL-10 during administration.

In conclusion, several observations support the hypothesis that intestinal microflora play a role at least in the perpetuation of IBD. Treatment with exogenous probiotics may enhance the concentration of protective bacteria in intestinal microflora and therefore may be of therapeutic benefit in patients with IBD and pouchitis.

Future research on probiotic bacteria needs to be centred on obtaining more precise information on the mechanisms by which probiotics exert their beneficial effects *in vivo*; this will provide a scientific rationale for the selection of the best probiotic strains to carry-out large, double-blind, controlled clinical trials.

Key references

- Campieri M, Gionchetti P. Probiotics in inflammatory bowel disease: new insight to pathogenesis or a possible therapeutic alternative? *Gastroenterology* 1999; 116: 1246-9.
- Gionchetti P, Rizzello F, Venturi A, Brigidi P, Matteuzzi D, Poggioli G, Bazzocchi G, Miglioli M, Campieri M. Oral bacteriotherapy as maintenance treatment in patients with chronic pouchitis: a double-blind, placebo-controlled trial. *Gastroenterology* 2000, in press.
- Rembacken BJ, Snelling AM, Hawkey PM, *et al*. Non-pathogenic *Escherichia coli versus* mesalazine for the treatment of ulcerative colitis: a randomised trial. *Lancet* 1999; 354: 635-9.
- Schaafsma G. State of the art concerning probiotic strains in milk products. *IDF Nutr Newsl* 1996; 5: 23-4.

Novel approaches in the treatment of gastrointestinal and liver disease: a look into the future.
Galmiche J.P., ed. John Libbey Eurotext, Paris © 2000, pp. 33-35.

Strategies against bacterial toxins in the gut: the case of *Clostridium difficile*

Ingo Just, Fred Hofmann, Harald Genth

Institut für Pharmakologie & Toxikologie der universität Freiburg, Freiburg, Germany

Clostridium difficile, a Gram positive anaerobic bacterium, has been identified in the 1970s as the causative micro-organism of the antibiotic-associated diarrhoea (CDAD) and the pseudomembranous colitis (PMC). It is now acknowledged as the major cause of nosocomial diarrhoea, being involved in about 25% of cases of antibiotic-associated diarrhoea and in about all cases of PMC. The clinical symptoms vary from mild diarrhoea to pseudomembranous colitis. The histological picture of the PMC is characterised by patchy epithelial necrosis up to epithelial ulcerations. The characteristic « pseudomembranes » are composed of mucus, fibrin, leukocytes and cellular debris. The chief risk factor for CDAD is the exposure to antibiotics. Especially broad-spectrum antibiotics are thought to alter the normal microflora of the gut thereby allowing colonisation and growth of *Clostridium difficile*. The normal microflora seems to create an environment which is restrictive for *Clostridium difficile* growth rather than to generate inhibitory factors. Second- and third generation cephalosporins, clindamycin, ampicillin and amoxycillin are associated with high risk for the development of CDAD whereas aminoglycosides, fluoroquinolones and ureidopenicillins have a low prospensity to induce CDAD.

Pathogenic strains of *Clostridium difficile* coproduce two protein toxins, the enterotoxin (toxin A) and the cytotoxin (toxin B) which are not secreted but released from sporulating bacteria. In animal models the toxins are able to induce all the symptoms of the CDAD, secretory diarrhoea, mucosal damage, and inflammation of the mucosa. Based on these findings, both toxins have been classified as chief pathogenicity factors of the CDAD. The leading toxin, according to animal models, is toxin A whereas toxin B effects are secondary; toxin B acts cytotoxically on sub-epithelial tissue after toxin A-induced damage of the colonic epithelium allows access of toxin B. However recent findings have led to the notion that both toxins contribute equally in human disease.

The toxins are single-chain proteins (MW ~ 300,000 Da) which enter their target cells through receptor-mediated endocytosis whereby the cell receptors are so far unknown. In the cytosolic compartment, they exhibit their cytotoxic activity by inactivating small GTP-binding proteins of the Ras-superfamily by mono-glucosylation.

The first step in the treatment of CDAD/PMC is the discontinuation of the antibiotic therapy. Mild and moderate forms spontaneously cease after discontinuation. If not and in the case of more severe forms, antibiotic therapy is needed to eradicate *Clostridium difficile* Metronidazole or vancomycin are the antibiotics of choice and given orally for about ten days. Vancomycin is not enterally absorbed and does exclusively act from the luminal side of the gut. In contrast, metronidazole is absorbed (thereby causing systemic side effects) and is secreted into the colon. This pharmacological property is the basis for the parental application of metronidazole in the treatment of severe PMC. Severe and debilitating diarrhoea, needs in addition to antibiotic therapy, the preservation of fluid and electrolyte balance. The anti-motility drugs, e.g. loperamide, should be used cautiously because there are case-reports of toxic megacolon after loperamide treatment of CDAD.

Vancomycin and metronidazole show high response rates up to 100% However, about 20% of patients successfully treated for a first episode will relapse. Patients who relapse are at risk for further relapses. The relapse rate does not depend on the antibiotic used and is not due to antibiotic resistance. Vancomycin and metronidazole also disrupt the colonic microflora and thereby preserving the conditions which predispose for infection with *Clostridium difficile*.

The *Clostridium difficile* toxins are the causative agents which induce diarrhoea, mucosal injury and inflammation. Through these mechanisms the toxins prevent re-establishing of the normal microflora which is a prerequisite to keep down *Clostridium difficile*. Furthermore, the toxins seem to be involved in the colonisation by the clostridia. Thus, blocking the activity of the toxins will be an essential step to allow physiological reconstitution of the colon. Theoretically, there are two possibilities to block toxin activity: (i) Inactivation or degradation of the toxins and (ii) the inhibition of cell entry.

The non-pathogenic yeast *Saccharomyces boulardii* has been reported to reduce the incidence of CDAD and to be also beneficial in the treatment of recurrent CDAD. However, *S. boulardii* therapy is an adjunct to the standard antimicrobial treatment. *S. boulardii* therapy is a widely used anti-diarrhoeic drug, however with poor documented efficacy. In the case of CDAD, the therapy with the yeast may be more rational because findings were reported that *S. boulardii* produce a protease which is capable of cleaving off the cell receptor of toxin A thereby preventing its cell entry. Furthermore, the protease degrades toxin A itself resulting in its inactivation. *S. cerevisiae* (the brewer's yeast) is distinct from *S. boulardii* and therefore cannot be considered as inexpensive alternative to *S. boulardii*.

A promising approach is the immunotherapy to inactivate the *Clostridium difficile* toxins by specific antibody neutralisation. Several reports indicate that patients suffering from CDAD and especially those suffering from recurrent or severe forms of CDAD have an impaired antitoxin response. Furthermore, a case report showed that intravenous antitoxin A/B immunotherapy led to rapid recovery of patients who did not adequately respond to the standard antibiotic therapy.

Several vaccination approaches in animal models, especially the hamster model, clearly have shown a benefit for the treatment of CDAD. Vaccine strategies employed should induce a protective anti-toxin response to prevent tissue damage at the mucosal surface. The strategy is thought to require the induction of a toxin-neutralising, secretory immunoglobin A-mediated response at mucosal surfaces to inhibit binding of toxin A to intestinal brush border. Therefore, intranasal immunisation of mice with the non-toxic binding domain of toxin A has been applied which generates in fact sufficient levels of toxin-neutralising IgA. However, the i.m. route of vaccine application results in serum anti-toxin antibodies conferring protection from death and diarrhoea. Thus, also serum anti-toxin antibodies play a role in the immunity of the toxin-mediated musocal disease. It seems that antibodies against the non-toxic binding domain of toxin A and toxin B are fully protective. Because both toxins are involved in the onset of the PMC in humans and the antibodies against the binding domain are not cross-reactive, vaccination must target both toxins.

Currently, two strategies are followed: 1) passive immunotherapy, based on orally administered anti-ToxinA/anti-Toxin B antibodies to treat recurrent and severe forms of CDAD; 2) active immunisation using peptides from both toxins as vaccine to prevent relapses. However, based on the finding that patients suffering from CDAD have a decreased immuno response to the toxins and non-toxin antigens, the passive immuno-therapy seems to be more promising.

The increasing incidence in CDAD, future antibiotic resistance against *Clostridium difficile* germs and problems in treating satisfactorily recurrent CDAD demands the development of alternative therapeutic strategies against CDAD.

Key references

- Boquet P, Munro P, Fiorentini C, Just I. Toxins from anaerobic bacteria: specificity and molecular mode of action. *Curr Opin Microbiol* 1998; 1: 66-74.
- *Clostridium difficile* infection. *J Antimicrob Chemother* 1998; 41: Suppl. C.
- Kelly CP, LaMont JT. *Clostridium difficile* infection. *Annu Rev Med* 1998; 49: 375-90.
- Kelly CP, Pothoulakis C, LaMont JT. *Clostridium difficile* colitis. *N Engl J Med* 1994; 330: 257-62.
- Kyne, *et al. N Engl J Med* 2000; 342: 390.
- McFarlane, *et al. JAMA* 1994; 271: 1913.
- Salcedo, *et al. Gut* 1997; 41: 366.
- Surawicz CM, McFarland. Pseudomembranous colitis: Causes and cures. *Digestion* 1999; 60: 91-100.

Inhibition of intestinal secretion

Michael J.G. Farthing

Digestive Diseases Research Centre, St Bartholomew's & The Royal London School of Medicine & Dentistry, London, UK

Diarrhoeal diseases have a major impact on morbidity and mortality worldwide, with as many as four billion cases of acute diarrhoea occurring each year. Intestinal infection is the most common cause of diarrhoea and is responsible for the deaths of 3-4 million individuals each year. The seventh cholera pandemic continues to produce high morbidity and mortality in many parts of the developing world including the Indian sub-continent, sub-Saharan Africa and some parts of Central and South America.

Most of the deaths from acute infectious diarrhoea result from loss of fluid and electrolytes leading to dehydration and acidosis. Thus, the majority of these deaths are avoidable providing fluid and electrolyte losses are replaced promptly. Oral rehydration therapy (ORT) with glucose-electrolyte solutions has transformed the management of acute diarrhoea but these solutions do not reduce diarrhoea and can paradoxically increase faecal output as the child is rehydrated. In addition ORT does not reduce the duration of the illness. These shortcomings of ORT can discourage the child's carer and lead to the discontinuation of ORS administration.

There is therefore a perceived need for the development of agents that will directly inhibit secretory processes in the intestine thereby reducing fluid and electrolyte losses and decreasing the requirements for their replacement.

Pathophysiology of acute diarrhoea

Acute infective diarrhoea is due either to (i) **increased intestinal secretion** which often occurs in the absence of intestinal injury following exposure to secretory enterotoxins or (ii) **decreased intestinal absorption** as a result of intestinal damage or inflammation. In some instances however, these mechanisms may co-exist. Enterotoxin mediated intestinal secretion such as that induced by cholera toxin or the *E. coli* enterotoxins is the form of acute diarrhoea that is likely to be most amenable to control by anti-secretory agents.

Cholera toxin (CT) is the prototype enterotoxin and its mechanism of action has been studied in great detail [1, 2]. Until recently the main focus of the action of cholera toxin has been on the enterocyte and the enzymic activity of the A_1 sub-unit of cholera toxin which is a nicotinamide adenine dinucleotide (NAD)-dependent ribosyl transferase which covalently links adenosine diphosphate (ADP)-ribose to guanine nucleotide-binding protein (G protein), which activates G_s, the catalytic unit of the enzyme adenylate cyclase. This leads to an increase in intracellular cyclic AMP which through a series of intermediate steps results in phosphorylation of the transmembrane chloride channel protein and opening of the channel which permits chloride ion secretion.

E. coli heat-labile toxins (LT1 and LT2) are a group of proteins that are closely related structurally, functionally and immunologically to CT [1, 2]. Like CT, *E. coli* LT has the A and B sub-unit structure and activates adenylate cyclase. Other bacterial enteropathogens produce LT-like toxins including *Camplylobacter jejuni*, *Salmonella typhimurium*, *Salmonella enteritidis*, *Aeromonas* sp. and *Plesiomonas* sp.

E. coli also produce a group of low molecular weight enterotoxins that are heat stable (ST). ST differs from LT and CT in that it activates guanylate cyclase with an associated increase in the intracellular cyclic guanosine monophosphate (cGMP). Heat stable toxins are also produced by other enteric pathogens including *Yersinia enterocolitica*, *Vibrio cholerae* non-O1 and enteroaggregative *E. coli* which produces enteroaggregative *E. coli* heat-stable toxin 1 (EAST-1).

Secretory diarrhoea may be enhanced by a variety of endogenous secretagogues including prostaglandins, 5-hydroxtryptamine (5-HT) and substance P [3]. Immunological mechanisms may also be important particularly IgE mediated hypersensitivity reactions such as local anaphylaxis in the gut. Mast cell products and neurotransmitters are also involved, particularly histamine, 5-HT, prostaglandins, leukotrienes, platelet activating factor and substance P.

The evolution of agents for the inhibition of intestinal secretion

For many decades there has been a search for agents that will inhibit intestinal secretion and thereby reduce stool volume and the volume of fluid required for rehydration. Astringents such as tannins and heavy metal salts, and opium derivatives have been known since the last century but even the synthetic opiates have relatively weak anti-secretory activity in the gastrointestinal tract. In 1980, Powell and Field published a list of potential anti-diarrhoeal drugs which included anti-inflammatory agents (salicylates, indomethacin) and a variety of neuroactive drugs (somatostatin, propranolol, phenothiazines, etc.) *(table I)* [4]. They also included enkephalins as potential anti-secretory agents and recognised the importance of the enteric nervous system as a potential target for anti-secretory activity. The enterocyte however remained a focus for anti-secretory agents, popular targets

Table I. Potential anti-diarrhoeal drugs. (From [4].)

A. Locally active	D. Neuroactive drugs
1. Glucose-electrolyte solutions	1. Catecholamines
2. Heavy metals: Bi^{3+}, Al^{3+}	2. Somatostatin
B. Anti-inflammatory	3. Propranolol
1. Glucocorticoids	4. Phenothiazines
2. Salicylates	5. Local anaesthetics
3. Indomethacin	6. Opiates and derivatives
C. Organic anions	a. Opium derivatives
1. Gallic acid (tannin)	b. Synthetic opiates
2. *d*-Galacturonic acid (pectin)	i. Diphenoxylate
3. Nicotinic acid	ii. Loperamide
	c. Enkephalins

being chloride and calcium channels, and the calcium binding protein, calmodulin. Although anti-secretory activity can often be detected in animal models or *in vitro*, clinical studies have generally produced disappointing results [5, 6]. During the 1980s and 1990s, the research direction changed away from the enterocyte itself and towards the role of the enteric nervous system in secretory and absorptive processes.

New anti-secretory drugs

Neuronal pathways have now been implicated in pertubations of intestinal transport associated with bacterial infection. There is increasing evidence that CT, LT and ST and *Clostridium difficile* toxin produce their secretory effects at least in part via a neuronal reflex arc.

Cholera toxin

Current evidence suggests that CT activates a neuronal reflex arc which involves a sensory afferent neurone which is probably cholinergic, an interneurone in the myenteric plexus which has substance P as the neurotransmitter and a secretory type 1 neurone which is likely to be VIPergic. There is also evidence that CT can release a variety of endogenous secretagogues including 5-HT, neurotensin and prostaglandins [7-12]. 5-HT released from enterochromaffin cells is thought to activate the afferent limb of the neuronal reflex by $5\text{-}HT_3$ and possibly $5\text{-}HT_4$ neuronal receptors. Interneurones appear to propogate the secretory effects of CT distally in the small intestine.

Confirmatory evidence that a 5-HT initiated neural secretory reflex is important in cholera comes from pharmacological inhibition studies in mammalian intestine [13-15]. However, the most profound inhibitory effects can only be achieved when a 5-HT antagonist is administered prior to exposure to CT. Human studies however, have produced conflicting results. The $5\text{-}HT_2$ receptor antagonist, ketanserin given in combination with the $5\text{-}HT_3$ receptor antagonist, ondansetron, failed to reverse cholera secretion, as did the $5\text{-}HT_3$ receptor antagonist, tropisetron [16]. The $5\text{-}HT_3$ receptor antagonist, alosetron increased basal sodium and fluid absorption but failed to significantly reduce secretion in a human model of cholera [17]. However, a recent study with the 5-HT$_3$ receptor antagonist, granisetron reversed fluid and chloride ion secretion to net absorption [18].

Similar studies in mammalian intestine have been performed with substance P antagonists and have again confirmed a role for this secretagogue and neurotransmitter in CT secretion [19]. Both a peptide and highly selective non-peptide substance P antagonist reduced CT fluid secretion in a dose-dependent manner, with a parallel reduction in sodium and chloride ion secretion in mammalian intestine [19, 20]. Unlike the 5-HT$_3$ receptor antagonist, granisetron, the substance P antagonists were not able to net reverse secretion to absorption.

The importance of VIP in CT-induced fluid secretion is also supported by inhibition studies. The VIP antagonist [4Cl-D-Phe [21], Leu [11]] VIP converted fluid secretion in rat jejunum to net absorption [22]. Similarly, the sigma receptor agonist, igmesine which reverses VIP-induced increases in short circuit current in mouse ileum mounted in Ussing chambers, reduced CT induced secretion in rat jejunum *in vivo* and was effective when given both before and following establishment of the secretory state [23].

These observations are entirely consistent with a neural reflex involving 5-HT neural receptors on an afferent sensory nerve, a cholinergic interneurone in the myenteric plexus and a secretory VIPergic neurone. These studies have clearly identified a number of potential novel targets for anti-secretory pharmacotherapy.

E. coli enterotoxins

LT has marked structural homogeneity with CT and is known to activate adenylate cyclase in enterocytes. LT however, does not release 5-HT from enterochromaffin cells in the small intestine and LT induced secretion is not inhibitable by 5-HT receptor antagonists [24]. Similarly, LT secretion is not inhibited by substance P antagonists although the sigma receptor ligand, igmesine does inhibit both CT and LT secretion. Despite these differences between CT and LT, the action of the latter is inhibited by hexamethonium and lignocaine which support the view that the ENS is involved in LT secretion. We have also recently shown that LT, like CT releases VIP, again indicating that the secretory neuronal afferent is a VIPergic nerve.

The secretory activity of ST also appears to involve the ENS since fluid secretion is inhibited by tetrodotoxin, lignocaine and hexamethonium [25], but like LT, 5-HT does not appear to be involved.

Potential anti-secretory agents for the future

The demonstration that 5-HT has an important role in triggering the neural reflex clearly identifies an important potential new target for pharmacotherapy. 5-HT$_2$, 5-HT$_3$ and 5-HT$_4$ receptors all appear to be involved as secretion is inhibited by specific antagonists at these receptors. However, the potential for using these targets for therapy in human disease currently appears to be limited for two reasons; (i) only CT (not LT or ST) has been shown to depend on 5-HT to activate the local neuronal reflex in the enteric nervous system and (ii) 5-HT antagonists could only be used prophylaxtically since they appear to have little or no effect once the secretory state is established. It is not entirely clear however, as to why this should be the case since 5-HT$_3$ receptors are present on both enterochromaffin cells and enteric nerves suggesting that the drug should be active in both modulating 5-HT release and in inhibiting its effect on the neuronal reflex.

Substance P antagonists appear relatively weak antagonists of CT induced secretion and are ineffective against *E. coli* LT and ST, thus limiting their clinical application in acute watery diarrhoea.

The sigma receptor angonist, igmesine however, inhibits both CT and the *E. coli* enterotoxins [26]. Sigma receptors are known to be present on nerves in the ENS and this would seem to be a potentially useful class of drugs to pursue for the treatment of secretory diarrhoea in humans.

New proabsorptive drugs

In addition to endogenous secretagogues within the gut mucosa and ENS, there are also endogenous absorbagogues. Somatostatin and its receptors are found throughout the alimentary tract and are known to be important in the physiological regulation of gastric and pancreatic secretion. The role of somatostatin in controlling secretory and absorptive processes in the intestine is less well defined. However, somatostatin is present in some intestinal neurones which are considered to be proabsorptive. There is therefore the potential to use somatostatin or one of the longer acting somatostatin analogues in the control of secretory diarrhoea [27-29].

Another important family of proabsorptive neurotransmitters in the ENS are the enkephalins. Enkephalinergic nerves have been identified extending to the basolateral membrane of enterocytes and enkephalins have been shown to have proabsorptive activity. Enkephalins decrease short circuit current and potential difference across isolated rabbit ileal mucosa. The effect is blocked by tetrodotoxin but not by adrenaline or atropine indicating a role for enkephalins as pre-ganglionic neurotransmitters within the gastrointestinal tract. Enkephalins appear to have their major effect through delta receptor activation which induces a selective increase in chloride absorption. Enkephalins have also been shown to reduce CT-induced small intestinal secretion, at least in part, by inhibiting adenylate cyclase through delta-opioid receptors.

The pro-absorptive, anti-secretory activity of endogenous enkephalins has been exploited in a major new drug development [30, 31]. Endogenous enkephalins are rapidly degraded by a membrane-bound metalloproteinase, enkephalinase. This enzyme is abundant in the gastrointestinal tract and accounts for over 85% of the hydrolysis of methionine- and leucine-enkephalins. A potent inhibitor of enkephalinase has been developed originally known as acetorphan but recently renamed, racecadotril. This agent has been shown to have anti-secretory activity against several secretagogues including CT and prostaglandins [32] and is effective in the clinical management of acute diarrhoea in both adults [33] and children [34]. This novel approach to the pharmacotherapy of secretory diarrhoea would appear to be promising and has a major advantage over standard opiate anti-diarrhoeal agents in that it does not produce entero-pooling and rebound constipation.

References

1. Rao MC. Molecular mechanisms of bacterial toxins. In: Farthing MJG, Keusch GT, eds. *Enteric infection*. London: Chapman & Hall, 1989: 87-104.
2. Field M, Fao MC, Chang EB. Intestinal electrolyte transport and diarrhoeal disease. *N Eng J Med* 1989; 321: 879-83.
3. Farthing MJG. Acute diarrhea: Pathophysiology. In: Gracey M, Walker-Smith JA, eds. *Diarrheal disease*. Vevey: Lippincott-Raven Publishers, 1997 (vol. 38): 55-71.
4. Powell DW, Field M. Pharmacological approaches to treatment of secretory diarrhoea. In: Field M, Fordtran JS, Schultz SG, eds. *Secretory diarrhea*. Bethesda, Maryland: American Physiological Society, 1980: 187-209.
5. DuPont HL, Ericsson CD, Mathewson JJ, Marani S, Knellwolf-Cousin AL, Martinez-Sandoval FG. Zaldaride maleate, an intestinal calmodulin inhibitor, in the therapy of travelers' diarrhea. *Gastroenterology* 1993; 104: 709-15.
6. Holmgren J, Grennough WB III. Reversal of enterotoxic diarrhea by chlorpromazine and related drugs. In: Field M, Fordtran JS, Schultz SG, eds. *Secretory diarrhea*. Bethesda, Maryland: American Physiological Society, 1980: 211-8.
7. Hubel KA. Intestinal nerves and ion transport: stimuli, reflexes and responses. *Am J Physiol* 1985; 248: G261-71.
8. Cassuto J, Fahrenkrug J, Jodal M, Tuttle R, Lundgren O. Release of vasoactive intestinal polypeptide from the cat small intestine exposed to cholera toxin. *Gut* 198; 22: 958-63.
9. Munck LK, Mertz-Nielson A, Westh H, Bukhave K, Beubler E, Rask-Madsen J. Prostaglandin E_2 is a mediator of 5-hydroxtryptamine induced water and electrolyte secretion in the human jejunum. *Gut* 1988; 29: 1337-41.
10. Beubler E, Kollar G, Saria A, Bukhave K, Rask-Madsen J. Involvement of 5-hydroxytryptamine, prostaglandin E_2 and cyclic adenosine monophosphate in cholera toxin-induced fluid secretion in the small intestine of the rat *in vivo*. *Gastroenterology* 1989; 96: 368-76.
11. Bearcroft CP, Perrett D, Farthing MJG. 5-hydroxytryptamine release into human jejunum by cholera toxin. *Gut* 1996; 39: 528-31.
12. Turvill JL, Connor P, Farthing MJG. Enterochromaffin cell 5-HT_3 autoreceptors inhibit cholera toxin (CT)-induced 5-HT release. *Gut* 1997: 41: A39.
13. Beubler E, Horina G. 5-HT_2 and 5-HT_3 receptor subtypes mediate cholera toxin-induced intestinal fluid secretion in the rat. *Gastroenterology* 1990; 99: 83-9.
14. Buchheit KH. Inhibition of cholera toxin-induced intestinal secretion by the 5-HT_3 receptor antagonist ICS 205-930. *Arch Pharmacol* 1989; 339: 704-5.
15. Mourad FH, O'Donnell LJD, Dias JA, Ogutu E, Andre EA, Turvill JL, Farthing MJG. Role of 5-hydroxytryptamine type 3 receptors in rat intestinal fluid and electrolyte secretion induced by cholera and *Escherichia coli* enterotoxins. *Gut* 1995; 37: 340-5.
16. Ehere AJ, Hinterleitner TA, Petritsch W, Holzer Petsche U, Beubler E, Krejs GJ. Effect of 5-hydroxytryptamine antagonists on cholera toxin-induced secretion in the human jejunum. *Eur J Clin Invest* 1994; 24: 664-8.
17. Bearcroft CP, Andre E, Farthing MJG. *In vivo* effects of the 5-HT_3 antagonist alosetron on basal and cholera toxin-induced secretion in the human jejunum: a segmental perfusion. *Aliment Pharmacol Ther* 1997; 11: 1109-14.

18. Turvill JL, Farthing MJG. Effect of granisetron on cholera toxin-induced enteric secretion. *Lancet* 1997; 349: 1293.
19. Turvill JL, Farthing MJG. Substance P (SP) antagonist inhibits cholera toxin but not *E. coli* enterotoxin-induced secretion. *Gastroenterology* 1999; 112: A414.
20. Turvill JL, Connor P, Farthing MJG. Action of non-peptide substance P antagonist CP 96 345, on cholera toxin and *E. coli* enterotoxin-induced secretion. *Gut* 1998; 42: A25.
21. Farthing MJG. Pathophysiology of infective diarrhoea. *Eur J Gastroenterol Hepatol* 1993; 5: 796-807.
22. Mourad FH, Nassar C. Vasoactive intestinal peptide (VIP) antagonism prevents cholera toxin (CT)-induced fluid secretion in rat jejunum. *Gut* 1997; 41 (Suppl. 3): A39.
23. Turvill JL, Kasapidis P, Farthing MJG. Inhibition of cholera toxin (CT)-induced jejunal secretion by the sigma ligand, igmesine. *Gastroenterology* 1999; 112: A414.
24. Turvill JL, Farthing MJG. Selective 5-hydroxytryptamine type 4 (5-HT$_4$) antagonist inhibits cholera toxin (CT) but not *E. coli* heat labile toxin (LT)-induced secretion. *Gastroenterology* 1996; 110: A368.
25. Eklund S, Jodal M, Lundgren O. The enteric nervous system participates in the secretory response to the heat stable enterotoxins of *Escherichia coli* in rats and cats. *Neuroscience* 1985; 14: 673-81.
26. Turvill JL, Kasapidis P, Farthing MJG. The sigma ligand, igmesine, inhibits cholera toxin and *Escherichia coli* enterotoxin induced jejunal secretion in the rat. *Gut* 1999; 45: 564-9.
27. Farthing MJG. The role of somatostatin analogues in the treatment of refractory diarrhoea. *Digestion* 1996; 57: 107-12.
28. Fried M. Octreotide in the treatment of refractory diarrhea. *Digestion* 1999; 60: 42-6.
29. Abbas Z, Moid I, Khan AH, Jafri SM, Shah SH, Abid S, Hamid S. Efficacy of octreotide in diarrhoea due to *Vibrio cholerae*: a randomized, controlled trial. *Ann Trop Med Parasitol* 1996; 90: 507-13.
30. Turvill JL, Farthing MJG. Enkephalins and enkephalinase inhibitors in intestinal fluid and electrolyte transport. *Eur J Gastro Hepatol* 1997; 9: 877-80.
31. Farthing MJG. Enkephalinase inhibition: a rational approach to anti-secretory therapy for acute diarrhoea. *Aliment Pharmacol Ther* 1999; 13 (Suppl. 6): 1-2.
32. Primi MP, Beuno L, Baumer P, Berard H, Lecomte JE. Racecadotril demonstrates intestinal anti-secretory activity *in vivo*. *Aliment Pharmacol Ther* 1999; 13 (Suppl. 6): 3-7.
33. Hamza H, Khalifa HB, Baumer P, Berard H, Lecomte JM. Racecadotril *versus* placebo in the treatment of acute diarrhoea in adults. *Aliment Pharmacol Ther* 1999; 13 (Suppl. 6): 15-9.
34. Turck D, Berard H, Fretault N, Lecomte JM. Comparison of racecadotril and loperamide in children with acute diarrhoea. *Aliment Pharmacol Ther* 1999; 13 (Suppl. 6): 27-32.

Novel approaches in the treatment of gastrointestinal and liver disease: a look into the future.
Galmiche J.P., ed. John Libbey Eurotext, Paris © 2000, pp. 45-58.

Multiple therapy in hepatitis C and hepatitis B

Yves Benhamou, Vlad Ratziu, Thierry Poynard

Service d'Hépato-Gastroentérologie, Groupe Hospitalier Pitié-Salpêtrière, Paris, France

The major hepatological consequence of hepatitis C virus (HCV) and hepatitis B virus (HBV) infections is the progression to cirrhosis and its potential complications: haemorrhage, hepatic insufficiency and primary liver cancer. Standard therapies have been established in chronic hepatitis C and B with an efficacy on virological endpoint as well as histological endpoints. For HCV the first approved therapy was interferon in monotherapy and then the combination of ribavirin with interferon. For HBV the first approved therapy was interferon, then vidarabin monophosphate and recently lamivudine. So far no combination regimen has clearly demonstrated a better efficacy. The aim of this article is to review the different treatments and their potential in association both for hepatitis C and B.

Hepatitis C

Efficacy of ribavirin interferon combination regimen in chronic hepatitis C
Efficacy of combination regimen on viral endpoints

When the 2 pivotal trials of ribavirin and interferon combination were combined, the database included 1,744 treatment naïve patients. At the end of treatment, the percentage of patients with undetectable HCV RNA is significantly higher in the combination groups, 51% (260/505) in the IFN-R 48 week, 55% (278/505) in the IFN-R 24 week, 29% (147/503) in the IFN 48 week, and 29% in the IFN 24 week (66/231) *(figure 1a)*. At the end of the follow-up, the percentage of patients with sustained undetectable HCV RNA is also higher in the combination groups 41% (205/505), 33% (166/505), 16% (82/503) and 6% (13/231) respectively, with significant differences between all these groups *(figure 1b)*.

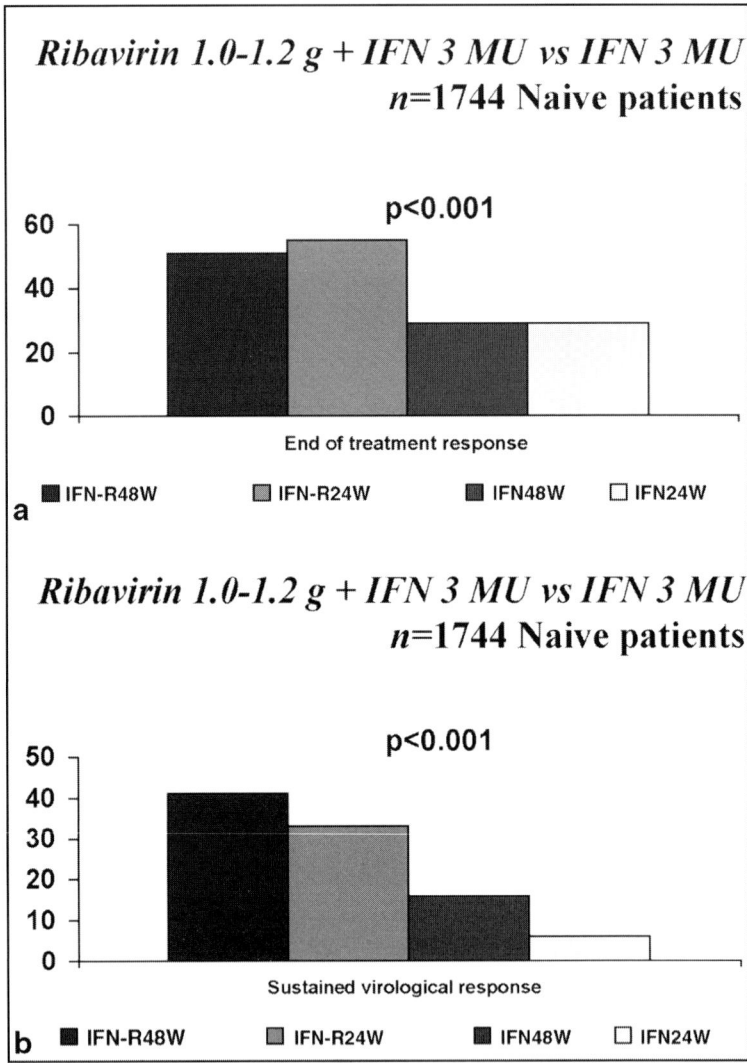

Figure 1. Efficacy of combination ribavirin-interferon at the end of the treatment (panel a) and at the end of 24 weeks follow-up (panel b). (From: Poynard, *Lancet* 1998; Hutschinson *N Engl J Med* 1998.)

These results demonstrate that there is a combination effect without duration effect on the end of treatment response and that there is both a combination effect and a duration effect on the sustained response.

Efficacy of combination regimen on transaminases (figure 2a and b)

There is a strong correlation between the impact of treatment on viral load and transaminases. However transaminases activity has a lower specificity for sustained response than viral load. Twelve percent of patients with normal ALT at the end of follow-up are PCR positive.

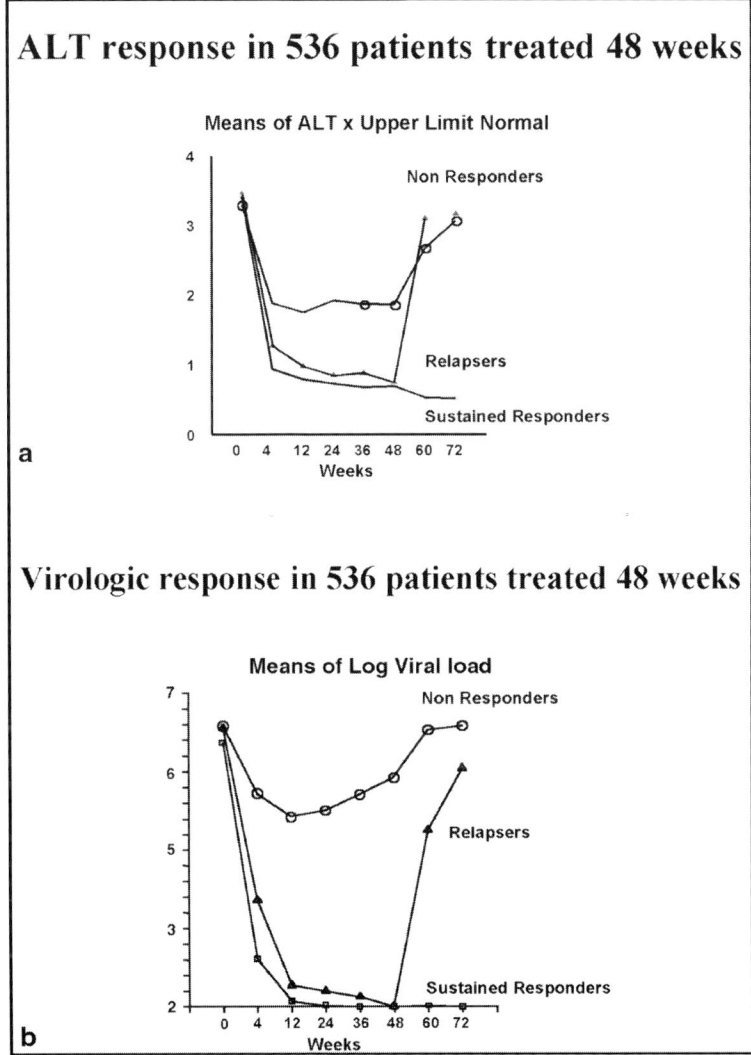

Figure 2. ALT (a) and viral response (b) to combination ribavirin-interferon.

Efficacy of combination regimen on histologic endpoints (figure 3a and b)

There is a significant improvement of activity grades and fibrosis progression rates when biopsies performed 24 weeks after the end of treatment is compared to baseline biopsies. Improvement is greater in sustained responders.

Efficacy of combination regimen on extra-hepatic manifestations and on quality of life

Little is known concerning the efficacy of treatment on extra-hepatic manifestation. During the treatment and because of the adverse events there is an impairment of health-related quality of life in comparison to baseline value. After the end of the treatment there is an

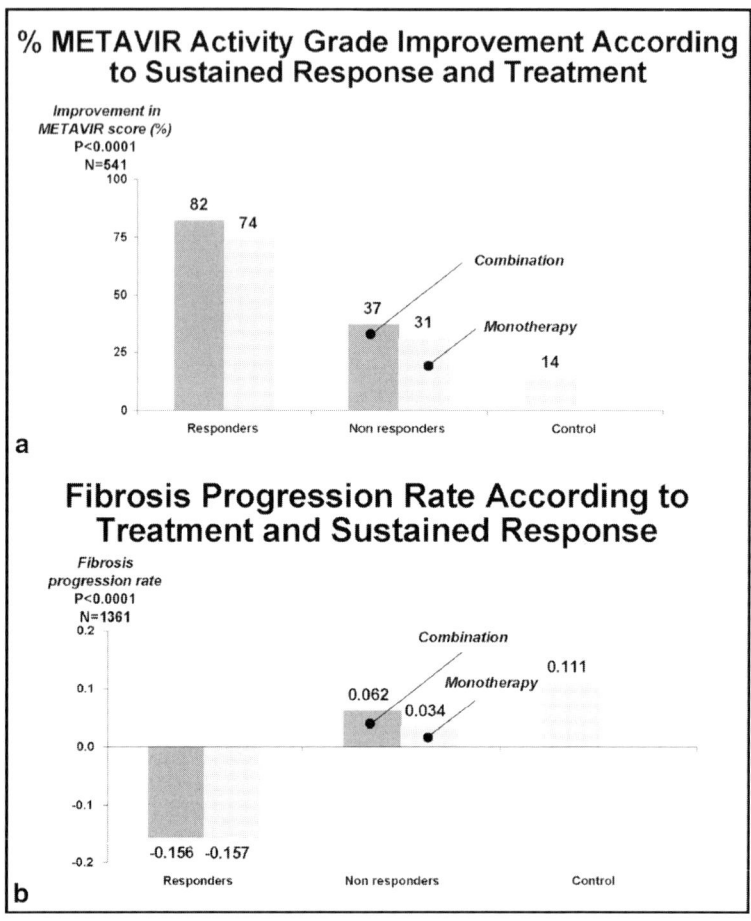

Figure 3. Improvement of histology after combination ribavirin-interferon. (a) activity grade, (b) fibrosis progression rate. (From Poynard et al. submitted.)

improvement of health-related quality of life in sustained responders in comparison to baseline level. In severe symptomatic cryoglobulinemia there is a clinical improvement by treatment.

Factors associated with treatment response and "à la carte" regimen *(table I)*

Careful analysis of pivotal trials has confirmed the independent prognostic values of five baseline characteristics. HCV genotypes 2 and 3 are associated with better response to the combination than other genotypes. For viral load, the ROC curves showed that there is no threshold that had either a positive or negative predictive value. Therefore, the simplest way to classify viral load into high or low is to take the median, which was 3.5 million copies. For age, the threshold of 40 years seems to have the best accuracy. Because the multivariate analysis showed that these 5 factors could only explain 20% of the variability of the sustained response, we need to identify the other independent factors. These

Table I. Sustained virologic response to different regimens according to baseline characteristics.

Baseline characteristics	IFN-Ribavirin 48w	IFN-Ribavirin 24w
Genotype		
2 or 3	65%	67%
1, 4, 5 or 6	30%	18%
Mean HCV RNA		
≤ 3.5 x 10^6 copies/ml	44%	40%
> 3.5 x 10^6 copies/ml	38%	26%
Age		
≤ 40 years	48%	40%
> 40 years	34%	26%
Fibrosis stage		
No or portal fibrosis	43%	36%
Septal fibrosis or more	36%	23%
Gender		
Female	46%	39%
Male	38%	30%
Combination of virological factors		
Genotype 2,3 ≤ 3.5 x 10^6	65%	71%
Genotype 2,3 > 3.5 x 10^6	65%	62%
Genotype 1, 4, 5, 6 ≤ 3.5 x 10^6	33%	26%
Genotype 1, 4, 5, 6 > 3.5 x 10^6	27%	10%
Combination of non virological factors		
Woman, ≤ 40 y, no or portal fibrosis	57%	56%
Men, > 40 y, septal fibrosis or more	34%	25%
Extreme favorable population		
Woman, ≤ 40 y, no or portal fibrosis Genotype 2, 3 ≤ 3.5 x 10^6 cop	79%	69%
Extreme unfavorable population		
Men, > 40 y, septal fibrosis or more, Genotype 1, 4, 5, 6 > 3.5 x 10^6	9%	8%

analyses have excluded that the kinetics of viral load at 4 and 12 weeks permit to take very early therapeutic decision.

There is no place for interferon monotherapy at a dose of 3 million units 3 times a week for either 24 or 48 weeks even in the most favorable patient.

Duration of combination regimen: 12, 24 or 48 weeks?

The first question is whether treatment can be stopped at 12 weeks in some subgroups because of a high probability of non-response. There was no consensus at the recent international conference. From our data this approach cannot be recommended because in the 48-week regimen, among the patients who had a positive PCR at 12 weeks, we observed a sustained response in 10% of patients. Even 24 weeks regimen induces a sustained response in 4% of these patients.

The choice of 24 or 48 weeks for combination therapy has been clarified. The crucial time to make this decision is at 24 weeks based on the results of HCV PCR testing. In patients who are PCR negative at 24 weeks (59% of the patients in these studies), the goal is to reduce the relapse rate. There was an overall highly significant improvement with 48 weeks of treatment (74% sustained responders) *versus* 24 weeks (59% sustained responders). Since patients with many favorable response factors benefit less from 48 weeks of treatment, consideration can be given to stopping at 24 weeks in these patients. A simple strategy could be to consider only the HCV genotype, and stop treatment at week 24 in genotype 2 and 3 responders, since the sustained response was 82% in patients treated 24 weeks *versus* 84% in patients treated 48 weeks. However, from our results it seems hazardous to recommend a strategy based only on virologic characteristics. There are in fact 5 independent response factors, and to take into account only one factor among these five is an over-simplification that could lead to errors in different populations or subgroups. For example, we have identified that patients with genotype 2 or 3 who are PCR negative at 24 weeks and who have extensive fibrosis will have a better sustained response with 48 weeks of treatment, 80%, compared to 65% in patients whose treatment is stopped at 24 weeks. For a population of older men with extensive fibrosis, the choice of 48 weeks duration in responders should not be based only on genotype and viral load. The recommendation of the international consensus conference to treat patients with genotype 2 or 3 for only 24 weeks, regardless of the other factors, seems inappropriate. Furthermore from a clinical point of view there is a risk to over simplify a decision according to a specific threshold, *i.e.* choice of 48 weeks treatment if the viral load is 3.75 millions and 24 weeks if 3.25 millions or 39 *versus* 41 years of age. This argues for taking the decision on both the number of independent factors and the tolerance to the combination.

Similarly, the recommendation of the international consensus conference to treat patients with genotype 1 for only 6 months if the level of viremia is low is not correct according to our results. This recommendation would lead to a reduction of 18% of the sustained response rate obtained by the 48-week regimen.

Suggested algorithm for the treatment (figures 4 and 5)

Finally, our recommendation is to treat naive patients with interferon ribavirin combination for 24 weeks and to test the HCV PCR at this point.

If HCV RNA is undetectable, the decision to continue the combination for 24 weeks or not should be taken according to the number of favorable factors. It seems reasonable to stop treatment in case of the presence of almost all the favorable factors, *i.e.*, 4 or five factors. For patients with less than 4 factors, who represented 46% of the population, its seems useful to continue the treatment for a total of 48 weeks.

For patients who remain PCR positive at 24 weeks the choice of whether to treat for 24 or 48 weeks has not been fully resolved. From the perspective of HCV eradication, the

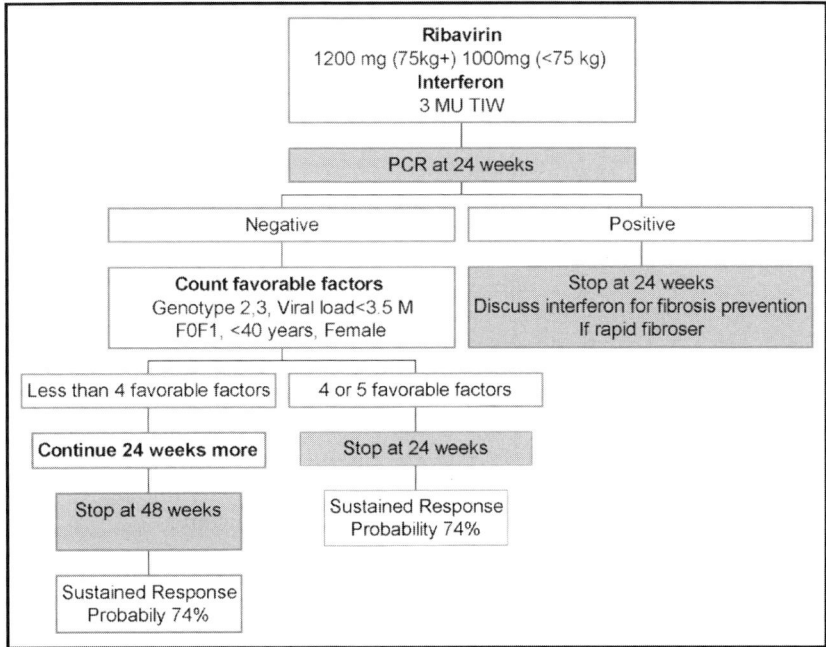

Figure 4. Proposed treatment regimen algorithm according to response factors.

combination can be stopped at 24 weeks, as the probability of obtaining a sustained virologic response is 2%. The remaining question concerns the usefulness of continuing the treatment in order to reduce histologic damage, since interferon and ribavirin have not only antiviral, but also antifibrotic and immuno-modulatory effects. Studies are needed to assess whether patients who fail to respond to combination therapy will benefit from either long-term interferon monotherapy or combination therapy.

Usefulness of genotype and viral load determinations

For patients who remain PCR positive after 24 weeks of IFN-R, there is no need to determine the genotype or perform any quantitative measurement before or during treatment. The combination can be stopped whatever the response factors. In contrast, for patients who are PCR negative at 24 weeks, clinicians need to know the genotype and the baseline viral load in order decide whether to continue treatment for an additional 24 weeks. ALT, PCR or viral load measurements at 4 or 12 weeks are not useful. However, for the very high risk group (men, older than 40 years and with at least septal fibrosis, F2) therapy should be continued whatever their viral characteristics.

Management of patients with cirrhosis *(figure 6)*

In patients with cirrhosis, ribavirin interferon combination achieved a sustained virologic response (below 100 copies per ml 6 months after the end of the treatment) in 20% by the combination *versus* 5% by interferon alone (p = 0.01).

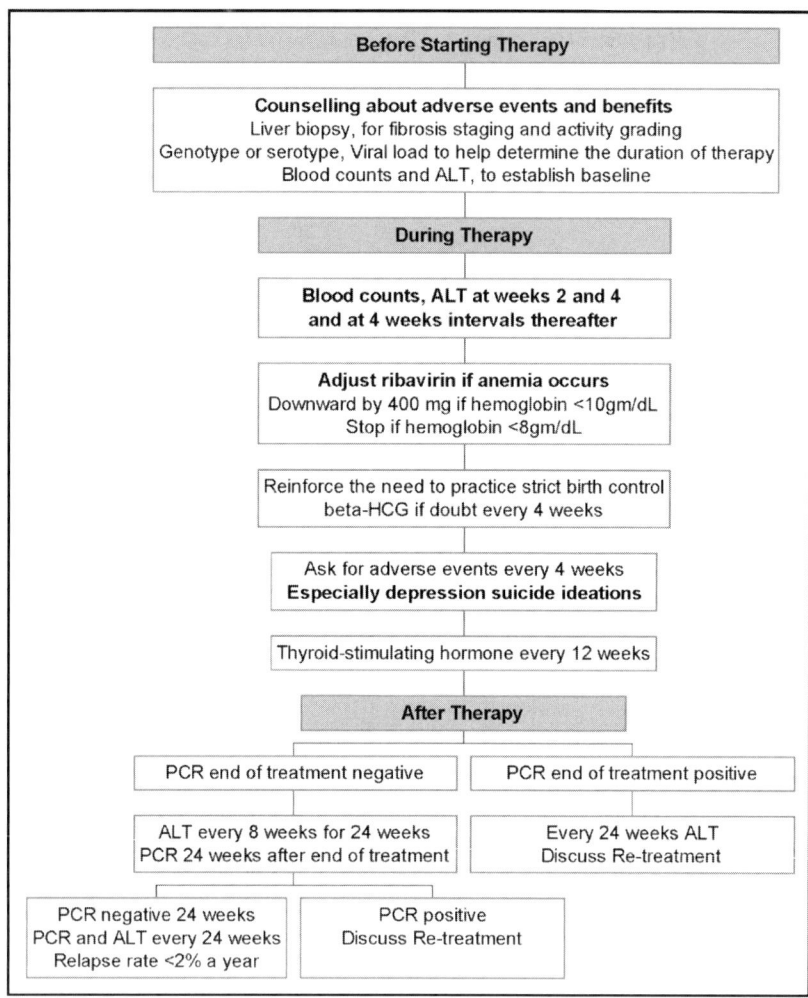

Figure 5. Proposed follow-up of treated patients.

Safety of interferon and ribavirin

Patients should be fully informed of the potential adverse events before starting therapy.

Severe adverse events

For interferon the main severe adverse events are depression, suicidal ideation, suicide and sustained hypothyroïdia. For ribavirin the main severe adverse events are anemia and teratogenic effects. There is a 3 gr/dl mean drop in hemoglobin concentration occurring in the first 4 weeks of treatment. Blood cell count must be checked at least 2 and 4 weeks after starting therapy and every 4 weeks there after. In case of hemoglobin lower than 10 g/dl ribavirin should be reduced by 50%. In case of hemoglobin lower than 8 g/dl ribavirin should be stopped.

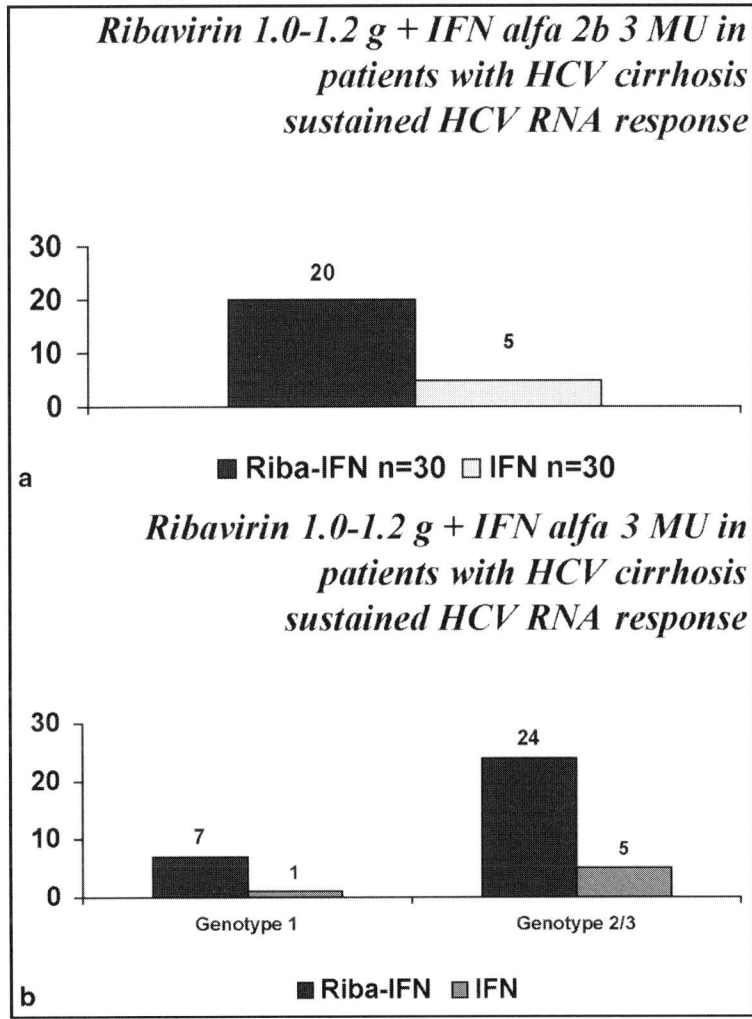

Figure 6. Efficacy of ribavirin interferon among patients with cirrhosis. Pivotal randomized trials (panel a) and pooled European database (panel b). (a) From: Poynard et al., Lancet 9151, 1999; (b) from: Schalm et al. Gastroenterology 1999; 117: 408-13.

Frequent adverse events

For interferon the most frequent adverse events are flu-like symptoms and alopecia.

For ribavirin the most frequent adverse events are anemia, and less frequently pharyngitis, insomnia, dyspnea, pruritus, rash, nausea and anorexia.

Contraindication to treatment

Contraindications to alpha interferon therapy include psychosis, severe depression, active substance or alcohol abuse, severe heart disease, severe neutropenia or thrombocytopenia, organ transplantation (except liver), decompensated cirrhosis, uncontrolled seizures, pregnancy, and non-reliable method of contraception.

Absolute contraindications to ribavirin are pregnancy, non-reliable method of contraception, hemodialysis, end-stage renal failure, severe anemia, and hemoglobinopathies. Relative contraindications are medical conditions in which anemia can be dangerous especially coronary heart disease and cerebrovascular disease. Fatal myocardial infarctions and strokes have been reported during combination therapy. Patients with a preexisting hemolysis or anemia (hemoglobin < 11 gm per dl) should not receive ribavirin.

Other multiple therapy in hepatitis C

Several drugs have shown non significant (Non steroidal anti-inflammory drugs) or marginal (ursodesoxycholic acid, glycyrrhizin, alpha-thymosin, interleukin 12) benefit alone or in association with interferon. The most promising drug as immuno-stimulating agent are HCV vaccine or dugs promoting a Th1/Th2 effect.

Waiting for a new generation of anti-viral drugs (anti-helicase, anti polymerase, anti-protease) there is also a place for anti-fibrotic drugs. Colchicine has sofar not demonstrated any effect. Sylimarin is presently in phase3 evaluation. Interleukin 10 is in phase 2 evaluation.

Pegylated interferon phase 3 trials are in progress, both in monotherapy or combined with ribavirin. The preliminary analysis of these trials suggest that a 10% increase of sustained response in comparison to standard interferon, could be achieved by these pegylated interferons, with an acceptable tolerability.

In conclusion, combination interferon alfa-2b plus ribavirin is the new first line treatment for chronic hepatitis C. It seems reasonable to recommend 48 weeks of treatment only for patients who are PCR negative at 24 weeks and who do not have 4 or 5 favorable response factors.

Hepatitis B

Interferon monotherapy was the first approved treatment in chronic hepatitis B *(figure 7, tables II and III)*. Vidarabin monophosphate was approved in few countries but had a bad risk-benefit ratio. Recently lamivudine has been approved in monotherapy *(figure 8, tables IV and V)*.

So far the different combination regimen investigated with alpha interferon have been disappointing, with marginal improvement or non significant effect: vidarabin, corticosteroid, HBV vaccine, gamma interferon, famciclovir, pencyclovir, levamisole, alpha-thymosin, and gamma interferon.

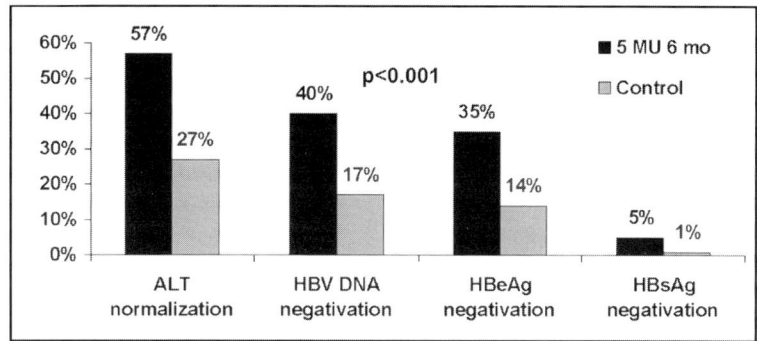

Figure 7. Meta-analysis: chronic hepatitis B IFN 5 MU 6 mo *vs* control. (Adapted from Wong *et al. Ann Intern Med* 1993; 119: 312-23.)

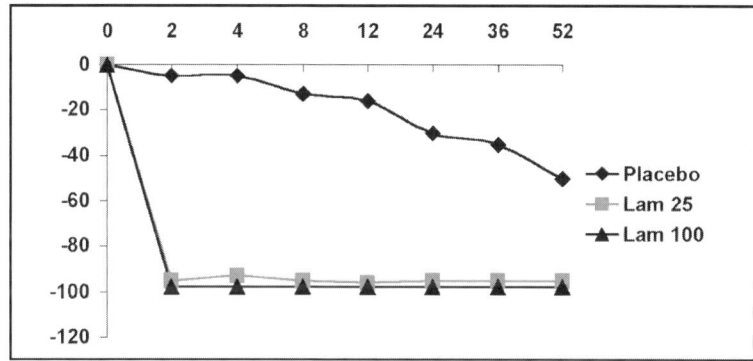

Figure 8. A one-year trial of lamivudine for chronic hepatitis B. (From Lai *et al.*, *N Engl J Med* 1998; 339: 61-8.)

Table II. Interferon advantages.

- Decrease of ALT, HBV DNA, HBeAg
- Decrease of necrosis and inflammation
- Decrease of fibrosis
- No mutation
- Few relapse after seroconversion

Table III. Interferon disadvantages.

- Adverse events
- Very slow improvement of ALT, HBV DNA
- Difficult to use in severe disease, transplanted, immunosuppressed
- No HBsAg seroconversion

Table IV. Lamivudine advantages.

- Minimal adverse events
- Rapid reduction of serum HBV DNA
- Decrease of ALT
- Decrease of necrosis and inflammation
- Decrease of fibrosis

Table V. Lamivudine disadvantages.

- Reverse transcriptase inhibitor with little effect on episomal template (closed circular DNA)
- No HBsAg seroconversion
- Incidence relapse even after Hbe seroconversion: non stop treatment?
- Incidence YMDD mutations: 100% 10 y?

According to the few published trials, the combination of lamivudine and interferon should be investigated further. A first phase 2 randomized trial (only 16 weeks) was disapointing. Another randomised clinical trial has compared combination in 230 predominantly Caucasian patients with hepatitis B e antigen (HBeAg) and HBV DNA positive chronic hepatitis B. Previously untreated patients were randomised to receive: combination therapy of lamivudine 100 mg daily with alpha interferon 10 million units three times weekly for 16 weeks after pretreatment with lamivudine for eight weeks (n = 75); alpha interferon 10 million units three times weekly for 16 weeks (n = 69); or lamivudine 100 mg daily for 52 weeks (n = 82). The primary efficacy end point was the HBeAg seroconversion rate at week 52 (loss of HBeAg, development of antibodies to HBeAg and undetectable HBV DNA). The HBeAg seroconversion rate at week 52 was 29% for the combination therapy, 19% for interferon monotherapy, and 18% for lamivudine monotherapy ($p = 0.12$ and $p = 0.10$, respectively, for comparison of the combination therapy with interferon or lamivudine monotherapy). The HBeAg seroconversion rates at week 52 for the combination therapy and lamivudine monotherapy were significantly different in the per protocol analysis (36% (20/56) v 19% (13/70), respectively; $p = 0.02$). The effect of combining lamivudine and interferon appeared to be most useful in patients with moderately elevated alanine aminotransferase levels at baseline. Adverse events with the combination therapy were similar to interferon monotherapy; patients receiving lamivudine monotherapy had significantly fewer adverse events. HBeAg seroconversion rates at one year were similar for lamivudine monotherapy (52 weeks) and standard alpha interferon therapy (16 weeks).

Finally several new drugs are in phase 2 and phase 3 evaluation: entecavir, adefovir, b-L-FD4C, L-FMAU, IL-12, HBV reinforced vaccine. An evaluation of the combinations between these drugs and interferon and lamivudine are also recommended.

Key references

Hepatitis C

- Consensus Statement. EASL International Consensus Conference on Hepatitis C. *J Hepatol* 1999; 30: 956-61.

- Davis GL, Esteban-Mur R, Rustgi V, *et al.* Interferon alfa 2b alone or in combination with ribavirin for the treatment of relapse of chronic hepatitis C. *N Engl J Med* 1998; 339: 1493-99.
- Hoofnagle JH. Therapy of viral hepatitis. *Digestion* 1998; 59 (5): 563-78.
- McHutchison JG, Gordon SC, Schiff ER, *et al.* Interferon Alfa 2b alone or in combination with ribavirin as initial treatment for chronic hepatitis C. *N Engl J Med* 1998; 339: 1485-92.
- Poynard T, Marcellin P, Lee S, *et al.* Randomised trial of interferon alpha 2b plus ribavirin for 48 weeks or for 24 weeks *versus* interferon alpha 2b plus placebo for 48 weeks for treatment of chronic infection with hepatitis C virus. *Lancet* 1998; 352: 1426-32.
- Poynard T, McHutchison J, Davis G, Esteban-Mur R, Goodman Z, Bedossa P, Albrecht J, and the FIBROVIRC Project Group. Impact of interferon alfa-2b and ribavirin on the liver fibrosis progression in patients with chronic hepatitis C. *Hepatology* 1998; 28: 497A.
- Poynard T, McHutchison J, Goodman Z, Ling MH, Albrecht J. Is an "à la carte" combination interferon alfa-2b plus ribavirin regimen possible for the first line treatment in patients with chronic hepatitis C? *Hepatology* 2000; 31: 211-8.
- Schalm SW, Weiland O, Hansen BE, *et al.* Interferon-ribavirin for chronic hepatitis C with and without cirrhosis: analysis of individual patient data of six controlled trials. Eurohep Study Group for Viral Hepatitis. *Gastroenterology* 1999; 117: 408-13.
- Ware JE, Bayliss MS, Mannocchia M, Davis GL. Health-related quality of life in chronic hepatitis C: impact of disease and treatment response. The Interventional Therapy Group. *Hepatology* 1999; 30: 550-5.

Hepatitis B

- Dienstag JL, Schiff ER, Wright TL, Perrillo RP, Hann HW, Goodman Z, Crowther L, Condreay LD, Woessner M, Rubin M, Brown NA. Lamivudine as initial treatment for chronic hepatitis B in the United States. *N Engl J Med* 1999; 341: 1256-63.
- Farhat BA, Marinos G, Daniels HM, Naoumov NV, Williams R. Evaluation of efficacy and safety of thymus humoral factor-gamma 2 in the management of chronic hepatitis B. *J Hepatol* 1995; 23: 21-7.
- Kruger M, Boker KH, Zeidler H, Manns MP. Treatment of hepatitis B-related polyarteritis nodosa with famciclovir and interferon alfa-2b. *J Hepatol* 1997; 26: 935-9.
- Musch E, Hogemann B, Gerritzen A, Fischer HP, Wiese M, Kruis W, Malek M, Gugler R, Schmidt G, Huchzermeyer H, Gerlach U, Dengler HJ, Sauerbruch T. Phase II clinical trial of combined natural interferon-beta plus recombinant interferon-gamma treatment of chronic hepatitis B. *Hepatogastroenterology* 1998; 45: 2282-94.
- Mutimer D, Naoumov N, Honkoop P, Marinos G, Ahmed M, de Man R, McPhillips P, Johnson M, Williams R, Elias E, Schalm S. Combination alpha-interferon and lamivudine therapy for alpha-interferon-resistant chronic hepatitis B infection: results of a pilot study. *J Hepatol* 1998; 28: 923-9.
- Schalm SW, Heathcote J, Cianciara J, Farrell G, Sherman M, Willems B, Dhillon A, Moorat A, Barber J, Gray DF. Lamivudine and alpha interferon combination treatment of patients with chronic hepatitis B infection: a randomised trial. *Gut* 2000; 46: 562-8.

Novel approaches in the treatment of gastrointestinal and liver disease: a look into the future.
Galmiche J.P., ed. John Libbey Eurotext, Paris © 2000, pp. 59-64.

Gene therapy for liver diseases

Jérôme Gournay

Service d'Hépato-Gastro-Entérologie, Hôtel-Dieu, Centre Hospitalier Universitaire de Nantes, Nantes, France

The normal liver is an attractive target for gene therapy because of the peculiar structure of its endothelium. Indeed, many fenestrations are normally present in the hepatic endothelium which makes this organ readily accessible to large molecules such as DNA fragments or recombinant viruses present in the blood. Recently, gene therapy has emerged as a potential new treatment of liver diseases, especially liver malignancies. A vast range of experimental data obtained in cell culture experiments and animal models have allowed the beginning of clinical trials.

Principles of gene therapy

The principle of gene therapy relies on the introduction of foreign genetic material encoding therapeutic protein in the nucleus of the cells that are to be treated [1]. Such a strategy requires that the therapeutic gene is correctly chosen and that efficient gene transfer vectors are available.

Initially, gene therapy was intended to cure various inherited disorders, for which the fundamental genetic defect has been identified and cloned and was based on the concept of gene replacement, which is the replacement of an abnormal copy of a gene by a functional one [2]. This method has many theoretical advantages and requires site-specific and homologous recombination. However, it is poorly efficient and so far only applicable to cultured cells. Consequently, most of gene therapy experiments are currently based on gene augmentation, which implies the transfer of a functionally normal copy into a cell in addition to the defective gene. The major limitation to successful gene therapy of inherited diseases resides in the efficiency of gene vectors to ferry the therapeutic gene in a sufficient number of target cells and ensure its proper expression for a prolonged period of time.

On the other hand, gene therapy is an approach for the treatment of acquired hepatic diseases, such as liver tumors. Cancer is a multifactorial disease and the cellular and genetic mechanisms that govern its appearance and development are partially or totally unknown. Three different strategies can be envisionned for gene therapy of liver tumors. The first one is an attempt to correct a genetic defect that is responsible for the acquisition of the malignant phenotype. It has been shown that some human tumors fail to express normal tumor suppressor genes or overexpress oncogenes [3]. It is therefore tempting to speculate that tumors could be cured by transferring a normal copy of the mutated gene involved in tumorigenesis to restore a normal phenotype into the tumor cell. This approach is hampered by the present difficulty to genotype each patient and also by the numerous mutations in various genes usually found in established tumors. The second one is the introduction into the tumor cells a gene coding for proteins which are able to trigger or enhance cell death. Numerous approaches have been developed in the past years. The most popular is the "suicide-gene" strategy in which a gene coding for an enzyme able to activate a harmless prodrug into a toxic metabolite is introduced directly into tumor cells. One example is the gene encoding the herpes simplex thymidine kinase (HSV-Tk). Its expression results in the conversion of ganciclovir, a nontoxic nucleoside, into its cytotoxic metabolite, ganciclovir triphosphate *(figure 1)*. Consequently cells that express the gene become sensitive to the prodrug exposure. The third one is based on the amplification of the immune response against the malignant cells through the introduction of a gene coding for a cytokine into the tumor cells or in their vicinity.

DNA delivery systems

Chemical vectors

The DNA molecule containing the therapeutic gene is compacted and protected from degradation by complexing it with proteins or lipids. These complexes, now termed lipoplex or polyplex depending on the composition of the chemical moiety (lipid *versus* protein), are designed to promote entry into the cell, delivery in specific cellular compartments and transfer the gene into the nucleus. The therapeutic gene needs to be administered repeatedly because the transfected DNA persists in episomes than can express the gene for a week or so.

Viral vectors

The general strategy to design viral vectors is to delete part or all of the virus genome to impair their replicative potential and replace it with the therapeutic gene that is to be transferred to the target cells. The resulting viruses are therefore replication-defective since they are unable to replicate in the infected cell [1]. Retroviral vectors have been the most used vectors for years in the field of liver gene therapy. Retroviruses allow the integration of their genetic material in the host genome. However they require target cell division for infection. The strategy for transferring genes to hepatocytes with retroviral vectors relies upon the availability of strategies to induce hepatocyte division before retroviral infection. The regeneration can be induced by surgical hepatectomy, chemical injury, infusion of various growth stimulating drugs or vascular occlusion. Adenoviral

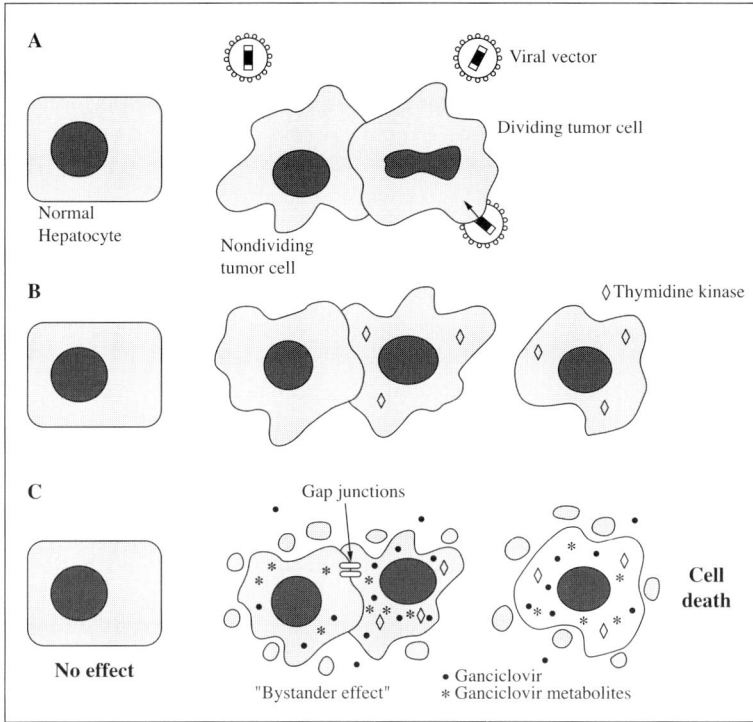

Figure 1. Suicide gene therapy. Tumor cells are transduced with the herpes simplex virus thymidine kinase gene. (a) Transgene expression in transfected cells results in synthesis of herpes simplex virus thymidine kinase, an exogenous kinase which can phosphorylate ganciclovir. (b) Systemic treatment with ganciclovir results in phosphorylation of the prodrug into toxic metabolites, resulting in cell death. (c) Transfer of toxic ganciclovir metabolites across gap junctions results in death of adjacent cells by the bystander effect.

vectors are able to infect quiescent cells such as hepatocytes in the normal adult liver. However, it soon appeared that transgene expression using these vectors is transient and most of the infected cells disappear rapidly after adenoviral infection.

Gene therapy for the treatment of inherited diseases of the liver

Liver directed gene transfer should theoretically be curative for inherited liver disesase. Crigler-Najjar syndrome type 1 is a congenital hepatic metabolic deficiency in bilirubin UDP-glucuronosyltransferase activity which leads to profound jaundice and death from kernicterus. The Gunn rat is an animal close to human Crigler-Najjar syndrome. Many experiments with Gunn rat have shown that the transfer of the UDP-glucuronosyltransferase gene into the liver cells led to a significant drops in serum bilirubin levels [4]. Retrovirus-mediated gene transfer of the fumaryl acetoacetate hydrolase gene, which defect is responsible for type I tyrosinemia, has been shown to induce a preferential repopulation of the liver parenchyma by the corrected cells [5]. Type I tyrosinemia might represent one particular disease in which gene transfer could be a preventive therapy against primary liver tumors. During the course of tyrosinemia, liver tumors often develop and represent an indication of liver transplantation.

Gene therapy for the treatment of hepatocellular carcinoma (HCC)

Many experiments *in vitro* have shown that gene transfer may be used for the treatment of HCC. Antitumoral cellular immunity can be induced after adenoviral delivery of the IL 2 gene in mice implanted in the liver with a syngeneic hepatocarcinoma cell line [6]. Similarly, retrovirus-mediated transfer of the tumor-necrosis-factor-α gene also induces an antitumor effect in mice subcutaneously implanted with another murine hepatocellular carcinoma cell line [7]. To ensure a specific expression of the transgene in primary hepatocellular carcinoma cells, many investigators have designed vectors harboring the transgene under transcriptional control of the regulatory region of the alpha-fetoprotein gene. In animal models in which primary liver tumors were generated in situ either in transgenic mice expressing a liver targeted oncogene or by feeding rats with a carcinogenic regimen, no real benefit of gene transfer was clearly demonstrated. In transgenic mice bearing SV40 T antigen or human hepatitis B virus envelope protein, a recombinant adenovirus bearing the p53 gene fails to suppress tumor growth [8]. The level of transfection of tumor cells obtained with either retroviral or adenoviral vectors was usually low [9]. One can hypothesize that this is due to the capillarization of the hepatic sinusoids during the course of hepatocarcinogenesis which results in the disappearance of the fenestrations present in the normal liver endothelium.

Gene therapy for the treatment of liver metastases

Due to the high predominance of liver metastases in various cancers and because such metastases are responsible for a large mortality, different groups have long tried to set up protocols for gene therapy of liver metastases. Using models based on intrahepatic as well as subcutaneous transplantation of tumor cell lines, a number of impressive results have been obtained and most transplanted tumors have been eradicated. Colon carcinoma metastases were efficiently treated with either retroviral or adenoviral vectors harboring the HSVTk gene. A true and effective systemic antitumoral immunity was achieved only after adenovirus-mediated transfer of cytokine genes such as IL2 and GM-CSF together with the HSVTk suicide gene [10]. This encouraging result prompted the initiation of a clinical trial aimed at treating colon carcinoma hepatic metastases [11]. Since tumor cells may be less infectable than their normal counterparts and because normal liver is highly sensitive to adenovirus-mediated gene transfer, such an original strategy might help to delineate a gene therapy protocole easily applicable in human patients.

Clinical trials

The first therapeutical gene transfer in humans is an approved protocol for correction of ADA deficiency which started in September 1990. Until October 1999, 380 clinical protocols including 3,173 patients have been done or are still in progress (according to the WEB site of the editor Wiley). Cancer therapy represents the largest proportion of both protocols (63.2%) and patients (68.3%). There are two protocols of treatment of hepatocellular carcinoma and 6 of treatment of liver metastases including 15 and 24 patients respectively. In a published trial, 15 patients with post hepatitis hepatocellular carcinoma were treated with percutaneous injections of wild-type p53 DNA-liposome complex [12]. Four patients experienced tumor volume reduction. No significant toxicity was reported.

Conclusion

After arousing great expectations, gene therapy for liver diseases has settled into a more humble and cautious phase of development. The treatment of inherited liver diseases required the long term expression of the transgene. The current vectors do not fulfil the requirements for such goal. Gene therapy for liver cancers is highly effective *in vitro* as shown in experiments using hepatoma cell lines. It is also effective in many *in vivo* models of liver tumors. However, severe limitations have been shown regarding gene therapy for HCC. Viral vectors are poorly effective for tumoral cell transduction. There is a need for relevant *in vivo* models of primary liver tumors. The situation is markedly different in liver metastases; there are now many lines of evidence that gene therapy might be effective in this setting.

References

1. Ferry N, Heard JM. Liver-directed gene transfer vectors. *Hum Gene Ther* 1998; 9: 1975-81.
2. Kay MA, Woo SLC. Gene therapy for metabolic disorders. *Trends Genet* 1994; 10: 253-7.
3. Bishop JM. Molecular themes in oncogenesis. *Cell* 1991; 64: 235-48.
4. Green RM, Gollan JL. Crigler-Najjar disease type I: therapeutic approaches to genetic liver diseases into the next century. *Gastroenterology* 1997; 112: 649-51.
5. Overturf K, Aldhalimy M, Tanguay R, Brantly M, Ou CN, Finegold M, Grompe M. Hepatocytes corrected by gene therapy are selected *in vivo* in a murine model of hereditary tyrosinaemia type I. *Nature Genet* 1996; 12: 458.
6. Huang H, Chen SH, Kosai K, Finegold MJ, Woo SL. Gene therapy for hepatocellular carcinoma: long-term remission of primary and metastatic tumors in mice by interleukin-2 gene therapy *in vivo*. *Gene Ther* 1996; 3: 980-7.
7. Cao G, Kuriyama S, Du P, Sakamoto T, Kong X, Masui K, Qi Z. Complete regression of established murine hepatocellular carcinoma by *in vivo* tumor necrosis factor alpha gene transfer. *Gastroenterology* 1997; 112: 501-10.
8. Bao JJ, Zhang WW, Kuo MT. Adenoviral delivery of recombinant DNA into transgenic mice bearing hepatocellular carcinomas. *Hum Gene Ther* 1996; 7: 355-65.

9. Ghosh SS, Takahashi M, Thummala NR, Parashar B, Chowdhury NR, Chowdhury JR. Liver-directed gene therapy: promises, problems and prospects at the turn of the century. *J Hepatol* 2000; 32: 238-52.
10. Chen SH, Chen XHL, Wang TB, Kosai KI, Finegold MJ, Rich SS, Woo SLC. Combination gene therapy for liver metastasis of colon carcinoma *in vivo*. *Proc Natl Acad Sci USA* 1995; 92: 2577-81.
11. Crystal RG, Hirschowitz E, Lieberman M, Daly J, Kazam E, Henschke C, Yankelevitz D, et al. Phase I study of direct administration of a replication deficient adenovirus vector containing the *E. coli* cytosine deaminase gene to metastatic colon carcinoma of the liver in association with the oral administration of the pro-drug 5-fluorocytosine. *Hum Gene Ther* 1997; 8: 985-1001.
12. Habib NA, Mitry RR, Sadri R. p53 and gene therapy for hepatocellular carcinoma. *Adv Exp Med Biol* 1998; 451: 499-504.

Pancreatic carcinoma: a challenge for the next century

Kaspar Z'graggen, Markus Wagner, Markus W. Büchler

Department of Visceral and Transplantation Surgery, University of Bern, Inselspital, Switzerland

Pancreatic cancer is an aggressive malignancy and radical surgery is the only curative treatment at present. Improvements in diagnostic imaging and advances in surgical technique led to an increase in resectability rates in centers with a high volume of pancreatic diseases. For cancer of the pancreatic head, pancreaticoduodenectomy is considered the standard procedure whereas distal pancreatectomy is performed for cancers of the pancreatic tail. Total pancreatectomy is indicated in the rare case of a tumor of the pancreatic body or in cases with tumor extension from the pancreatic head towards the body and tail of the gland. The pylorus preserving pancreatoduodenectomy (PPPD) is a more conservative variation of the classic Whipple procedure. The advantages of the PPPD are the preservation of gastric function to improve postoperative weight gain and quality of life without compromising radicality.

Scientific evidence for the superior function of PPPD over the classic Whipple procedure is currently not available, but the results of a prospective randomized study from our department are currently awaited.

Morbidity and mortality after pancreatic surgery have declined over the last two decades and mortality rates below 5% should be the standard in specialized centers. Although the improvement of long-term survival rates after radical resection of pancreatic cancer is less dramatic, recent studies from high volume centers report actual 5-year survival rates of 20-25% in non-selected patient groups. The role of palliative surgery in pancreatic cancer patients is controversial. Although several randomized trials seem to indicate that endoscopic stenting has a lower mortality than surgical bypass, recent series on biliary bypass for pancreatic cancer reported a mortality rate < 2%. In addition to the biliary bypass, surgery allows a gastric bypass during the same procedure, a policy that has been supported by one randomized study. Palliative pancreatoduodenectomy has also been proposed and may merit further discussion as mortality rates decrease and new adjuvante forms of treatment evolve.

In our surgical department 287 consecutive patients with pancreatic cancer have been treated between 11/93 and 12/99. Resectability was 58%, 25% and 17% of patients received a surgical bypass or underwent an explorative laparotomy. Resection consisted of classic pancreatoduodenectomy in 26%, PPPD in 43%, total pancreatectomy in 11% and pancreatic left resection in 10%. Mortality was 3%, surgical morbidity 27%, and the reoperation rate 4%. Tumor recurrence developed in 67% of patients after a median of 15 months. Calculated 5-year survival was 23% after a median follow-up period of 37 months. Surgical bypass was usually performed as a combined biliary and gastric procedure (58%), biliary bypass in 21% and gastric bypass in 19%. Mortality and morbidity after bypass procedures was 1.5% (1/67) and 18%, median survival 5 months.

The value of adjuvante radio/chemotherapy is still controversial. While one prospective randomized study demonstrated a survival benefit, the soon to be published ESPAC results, which enrolled more than 500 patients, will indicate future investigational strategies in the adjuvant treatment of pancreatic cancer.

In conclusion, resection for pancreatic cancer can be performed safely as a result of improved surgical techniques, perioperative management and probably centralization of these patients in specialized treatment centers. Actual data indicate, that for patients with pancreatic cancer a long-term survival of 20% or more is possible with radical surgery alone. To improve staging strategies, define the extent of lymph node dissection, the role of vascular resection and reconstruction and the place of palliative procedures will be some of the formidable challenges for the next years. Future research will improve the understanding of pancreatic cancer biology and novel therapeutic strategies such as immunotherapy or gene therapy in combination with modern surgery may bring hope for our future patients.

Key references

- Büchler MW, Friess H, Wagner M, Kulli C, Wagener V, Z'graggen K. Pancreatic fistula after pancreatic head reserction. *Br J Surg* 2000; 87: in press.
- Pedrazzoli S, DiCarlo V, Dionigi R, Mosca F, Pederzoli P, Pasquali C, Kloppel G, Dhaene F, Michelassi F. Standard versus extended lymphadenectomy associated with pancreatoduodenectomy in the surgical treatment of adenocarcinoma of the head of the pancreas: a multicenter, prospective, randomized study. Lymphadenectomy Study Group. *Ann Surg* 1998; 228: 508-17.
- Sener SF, Fremgen A, Menck HR, Wichester DP. Pancreatic cancer: a report of treatment and survival trends for 100,313 patients diagnosed from 1985-1995 using the national cancer database. *J Am Coll Surg* 1999; 189: 1-7.
- Warshaw AL, Pancreatic surgery. A paradigm for progress in the age of the bottom line. *Arch Surg* 1995; 130: 240-6.

Photodynamic therapy

Liebwin Gossner

Second Medical Department, Wiesbaden Hospital, Wiesbaden, Germany

The idea of treating tumors by photosensitizers is as old as the early 1900's. But reports concerning intraluminal photodynamic therapy in the gastrointestinal tract first began to appear in the late 1980s, and were greeted with both enthusiasm and controversy. In that respect, little has changed even today. It is not that photodynamic therapy (PDT) has been outdated, nor that its technical potential has been fully exhausted, nor that it has been superseded by more modern procedures. On the contrary, PDT is still going through a dynamic process of development, improvement, and standardization.

Photodynamic principle

Photodynamic therapy represents a minimally invasive, organ-preserving therapeutic modality. PDT involves three separate components: light, oxygen and a photosensitizing drug. PDT exploits the physical phenomenon that light is able to activate phototosensitizing compounds that are incorporated by tissue. Light energy which is absorbed by the photosensitizer is transferred in several steps primarily to oxygen within the tissue and leads to tumor destruction through oxydation processes. Laser light with a specific wavelength lying within the relative maximum of the absorption band of the applied photosensitizer is delivered endoscopically, through a flexible fiber, into the gastrointestinal tract, and is then used for topical irradiation of the sensitized dysplastic or malignant tissue.

Palliative treatment

Palliative treatment of stenotic tumors of the esophagus, stomach, and colon does not provide any hopeful prospects for widespread use of photodynamic procedures, either. Although a multicenter American study for obstructing esophageal cancer showed that fewer treatment sessions were required with PDT in comparison with Nd:YAG laser therapy, and that there was also a lower perforation rate, the economic arguments are not convincing here in view of the high cost of PDT and the short life expectancy in this group of patients [1]. The American health authorities have approved PDT exclusively for palliation, but in clinical reality there are in fact simpler thermodestruction procedures, and particularly in the esophagus, mature techniques using self-expanding metal endoprostheses are available for simpler and more effective palliation.

With regard to the palliative treatment of malignant stenoses of the bile ducts using PDT, one complete paper and one abstract have been published, reporting small numbers of cases. However, these require confirmation in larger studies-preferably multicenter prospective and comparative ones-before this treatment procedure can be seriously recommended [2]. Nor is PDT likely to be of any significance in the treatment of villous rectal adenomas and flat papillary adenomas, due to the alternative treatment procedures that are available and the low numbers of cases.

Curative treatment

Barrett's esophagus

The most frequent indication for PDT in the future may be Barrett's esophagus. However, PDT of any type is also in competition with the various methods of thermoablation and endoscopic mucosal resection (EMR) as well. The incidence of the diagnosis of Barrett's esophagus has rapidly increased in recent years. There is nowadays also a broad awareness of the metaplasia-dysplasia-carcinoma sequence, and this in part explains the increasing rate of diagnosis. In a more detailed discussion, it is useful to distinguish between Barrett's metaplasia with or without dysplasia on the one hand, and severe dysplasia or early Barrett's carcinoma on the other. The precondition for local endoscopic therapy for Barrett's esophagus with or without mild dysplasia should be that the method used allows complete ablation of the undesirable epithelium and complete restitution of orthotopic epithelium. The existing data do not yet allow firm conclusions to be drawn. However, the data on the use of PDT in the treatment of Barrett's epithelium seem to be lightly better in comparison with those for thermoablation [3-6]. In addition, ablation using the spot effects of thermal procedures – whether laser coagulation or thermocoagulation – produces varying depths and not infrequently causes tissue destruction that also affects the submucosa. By contrast, PDT with ALA is limited in its destructive effects on the mucosa, as has been adequately shown in animal experiments. In this respect, ALA-PDT has a clear advantage over thermocoagulation procedures. In addition, suitable light applicators can be used to achieve homogeneous and circumferential irradiation in a single session, over a length of up to 8 cm [7]. Summing up, it appears that ALA-PDT treatment of Barrett's mucosa with or without mild dysplasia has basic advantages over the alternative procedures, although there is still a lack of adequate clinical confirmation. In addition, it has not been adequately confirmed whether ablation techniques in general do in fact provide an economically defensible form of carcinoma prevention.

Although the case numbers concerned are smaller, the question of how to deal with Barrett's epithelium and severe dysplasia or early carcinoma is of much greater clinical relevance. The gold standard is undoubtedly still radical surgery, with partial gastric and esophageal resection. However, careful study of the published surgical data shows that there are good arguments for local therapy. On the one hand, there are the considerable morbidity and mortality rates associated with radical surgery, which even in high-grade dysplasia or early carcinoma in Barrett's esophagus amount to between 30% and 50%, or 3% and 5% respectively. The available surgical and pathoanatomical data indicate that the risk of lymph-node metastasis in high-grade dysplasia and in mucosal early carcinoma is almost zero. In any case, it is lower than the mortality rates with surgery. In choosing a local treatment procedure, endoscopic mucosal resection is undoubtedly the first option. However, EMR can only be used if the malignant lesions can be clearly located. In addition, the resection cannot exceed a certain size, and in multifocal conditions, too, EMR is not yet a suitable form of primary therapy [8]. This suggests one potential indication for PDT; whenever a biopsy has demonstrated malignancy or severe dysplasia but macroscopic identification is unclear, and in cases of long Barrett's segments with advanced histological changes, PDT should be considered as a primary form of local treatment.

With the usual form of PDT, strictures occurred in up to half of the patients, but all of these were easy to treat endoscopically. In Overholt's group, this relatively aggressive form of treatment was followed by complete remission in all patients, and this was also confirmed during a follow-up period of up to five years [5]. Using the "milder" form of ALA-PDT, which is limited to selective destruction of the mucosa, Barr's group and our own group achieved long-term complete remission in all cases of high-grade dysplasia. Long-term remission was seen in only around 75% of patients who already had early carcinoma, however [6]. When the mucosa has thickened by more than 2 mm, *i.e.*, when mucosal changes are already visible macroscopically, ALA-PDT is very likely to be inadequate, and a more intensive form of PDT should be used instead – for example, with mTHPC as the photosensitizer. The data on PDT in severe dysplasia and early carcinoma in Barrett's esophagus are very promising, but due to the small numbers of patients overall and the very short follow-up period, a conclusive assessment of the value of the method is not yet possible.

Early esophageal cancer

With regard to the use of PDT in the treatment of early squamous-cell carcinoma in the esophagus, there have also only been very few reports so far, at least from the Western hemisphere. When ALA is used as the photosensitizer, all of the patients with high-grade dysplasia who were treated in our group experienced complete remission, but only about half of those with confirmed early carcinoma had remissions. No significant side effects of the treatment were observed [9]. By contrast, the results of PDT with mTHPC of the

Lausanne group were better with regard to complete remission, although this was as the expense of increased morbidity. Summing up, PDT may therefore be of significance in the future for the treatment of high-risk patients with early squamous-cell carcinoma, since in comparison with radical surgery or aggressive chemoradiotherapy, PDT represents a form of minimally invasive treatment. Here, too, however, the search for optimal irradiation conditions is not yet complete.

Early gastric cancer

In Western countries, early gastric carcinoma is being diagnosed endoscopically with increasing frequency, and patients are receiving local curative treatment (and not only in inoperable cases). When prior staging examinations are carried out, the histological and endoscopic ultrasound findings can be used to identify with a high degree of certainty those patients able to benefit from local curative treatment. Particularly when endoscopic mucosal resection is not possible or is not successful, PDT represents a good alternative [10]. In our group at least the photosensitizer meta-tetrahydroxyphenylchlorin (mTHPC) has proved its value. With no significant morbidity and in particular with no cases of perforation, complete tumor destruction was achieved in ca. 80% of patient treated; The follow-up period is clearly limited, and the results achieved are therefore preliminary. Particularly in tumors that cannot be clearly located endoscopically ("biopsy carcinoma"), photodynamic treatment of larger areas using mTHPC – or even with ALA, which is much less problematic in clinical practice – is a procedure that is fundamentally different from thermoablation methods and mucosectomy, and should therefore be considered as a potential treatment option.

In conclusion, PDT is a fascinating concept, which will continue to occupy many research groups around the world in the coming years. Although a widespread clinical application for the method has not yet emerged, there are good prospects that PDT will be able to establish itself at major gastroenterological centers as an endoscopic procedure with few or no side effects in the treatment of Barrett's esophagus (high-grade dysplasia and early carcinoma) and, in selected cases, also for the treatment of early squamous-cell carcinoma and clearly gastric carcinoma.

References

1. Lightdale CJ, Heier SK, Marcon NE, *et al*. Photodynamic therapy with porfimer sodium versus thermal ablation therapy wit ND:YAG laser for palliation of esophageal cancer: a multicenter randomized trial. *Gastrointest Endosc* 1995; 42: 507-12.
2. Ortner A, Ernst H, Lochs H. Photodynamic therapy of malignant common bile duct stenoses. *Gastroenterology* 1998; 114: 9-14.
3. Gossner L, May A, Stolte M, Seitz G, Ell C. KTP-laser destruction of dysplasia and early cancer in columnar-lined Barrett's esophagus. *Gastrointest Endosc* 1999; 49; 8-12.
4. Laukka MA, Wang KK. Initial results using low-dose photodynamic therapy in the treatment of Barrett's esophagus. *Gastrointest Endosc* 1995; 42: 59-63.

5. Overholt BF, Panjehpour M. Photodynamic therapy for Barrett's esophagus: clinical update. *Am J Gastroenterol* 1996; 91: 1719-22.
6. Gossner L, Stolte M, Sroka R, *et al.* Photodynamic ablation of high-grade dysplasia and early cancer in Barrett's esophagus by means of 5-aminolevulinic acid. *Gastroenterology* 1998; 114: 448-55.
7. Gossner L, Sroka R, Ell C. A new long-range through-the-scope balloon applicator for photodynamic therapy in the esophagus and cardia. *Endoscopy* 1999; 31: 370-6.
8. Ell C, May A, Gossner L, *et al.* Endoscopic mucosal resection of early cancer and high-grade dysplasia in Barrett's esophagus. *Gastroenterology* 2000; 118: 670-7.
9. Gossner L, May A, Sroka R, Stolte M, Hahn EG, Ell C. Destruction of high-grade dysplasia and early carcinoma of the esophagus after oral administration of 5-aminolevulinic acid. *Cancer* 1999; 86: 1921-8.
10. Ell C. Gossner L, May A, *et al.* Photodynamic therapy of early gastric cancer with mTHPC. *Gut* 1998; 43: 345-9.

Laparoscopic surgery in the next century

Lars R. Lundell

Department of Surgery, Sahlgren's University Hospital, 413 45 Gothenburg, Sweden

Laparoscopic operations have grown rapidly in the popularity because of their beneficial impact on early patient recovery and reduction of postoperative pain. The promise of this new surgical approach led to many innovative laparoscopic adaptations of traditional open operations. Some of these are destined to become integrated into every day surgical practice, whereas others will be remembered as quaint technical tours de force.

Many if not most operations on the gastrointestinal tract and intra-abdominal solid organs, which formally require laparotomy, can now be performed laparoscopically. Laparoscopic cholecystectomy and antireflux operations are standard procedures, other operations such as laparoscopic colectomy for benign conditions, appendectomy and splenectomy are performed at many centres but have not yet moved into the main stream. More exotic laparoscopic exercises such as hepatic and pancreatic resections are performed at few centres but seem less lightly to achieve wide application in the near future. Laparoscopic treatment for potentially curable cancer is investigational and should only be done in a rigorous protocol setting.

The laparoscopic revolution began about ten years ago and has profoundly changed the way that surgeons, physicians and patients approached the treatment of certain diseases. We have now moved from a revolutionary to an evolutionary situation. Rapid changes have given way to careful study and critical evaluation. Nearly a decade of experience has now shown that laparoscopic operations benefit many patients and are associated with no greater risk than their traditional predecessors. Ongoing and future trials will determine which of the laparoscopic operations now being performed deserve to be continued.

The impact of laparoscopy on cancer management

Although the ultimate challenge for the reduction in cancer death is to prevent the neoplastic cell from developing and replicating, technical innovations have impact in both the timing of identification and the stage of cancer when discovered. Newer modalities involving alternatives to traditional radiological imaging, introduction of tumor markers and use of combinations of technologies are applied to management of our cancer patients with ever increasing expectations of facilitating the earliest possible recognition of a cancerous process. To evaluate laparoscopy in a scientific manner both as a diagnostic and therapeutic instrument in cancer care is the next challenges in the field of surgical endoscopy. During the last years studies have supported the use of preoperative laparoscopic assessment in patients diagnosed with oesophageal, gastric pancreatic and hepatobiliary malignancies. The goal of these studies is to identify subset of patients who might benefit from non-exstirpative approaches as offered by newer stent technologies as well as chemoradiation. An additional goal has been to offer staging technique that allows us to select patients who might benefit from neo-adjuvant therapy prior to tumor excision.

As a therapeutic tool for cancer management a laparoscope in approach has a particular interest in the treatment of cancer of the colon and rectum. Adequate margin of resection, nodal dissection and anastomotic creation have been reported. Besides technical consideration the extent of patients related benefits has to be further outlined. Clinical trials are ongoing which are designed to answer the ultimate question relating to cancer-free survival following the laparoscopic approach. It remains important to consider traditional open colonic resection as the "Gold Standard" but different endoscopic procedures will definitely emerge and develop within this field of abdominal surgery.

Transanal endoscopic microsurgery has emerged as a minimally invasive means of resecting rectal tumors. This is an endoluminal, minimally invasive technique that permits transanal excision of rectal lesions up to about 20 cm without a requirement of major abdominal operations. A full resection device has been developed from the model of the circula stapler used in surgical procedures to allow a completely endo-luminal transanal approach for resection of high risk polyps within the rectum and colon without requiring open surgery. In conjunction with the flexible endoscope this endoluminal resection devices use grasp but normal colorectal tissue and pulled into an open chamber which is then closed, staples fired and the knife blad brought behind staple line to effect the transmural resection. The full thickness resection devise use is similar to the transanal endoscopic micro surgery procedure but is less complex, less costly and the future will not require surgical environment to perform.

An increasing awareness has emerged in terms of minimal invasive techniques for gastric and early upper GI cancers. Interventional flexible endoscopic treatment, laparo-endoluminal resections, transgastrostomal endoscopic surgery and laparoscopic gastric resection (totally laparoscopic, laparoscopically assisted and hand assisted). The intervention of flexible endoscopic approach will be suitable for superficial early gastric cancer not involving the submucosa and the techniques include mucosectomy (submucosal resection) after epinephrine-saline injection into the submucosal layer and for instance laser ablation. The laparo-endoluminal mucosectomy is an alternative to this procedure and is particularly suitable for lesions in the posterior wall of the stomach and fundus. In these situations the laparoscopic surgeon and the skilled endoscopist work together. Another surgical approach is the transgastrostomal endoscopic surgery which is particularly useful for instance posterior wall lesions and it avoids the need for CO^2 insufflation. This technique can be used for both mucosectomy and local excisions. Wedge resections without lymphadenectomy may be adequate for smaller superficially lesions without significant submucosal involvement.

Intraoperative endoscopy is essential for locating the exact sight of gastric intraluminal muscle tumors for instance. For large exophytic lesions some recommend a two step approach that is endoscopic debalcing followed by laparoscopic resection.

The introduction of devices that allow insertion of the surgeons non dominating hand into the peritoneal cavity without loss of the pneumo peritoneum has greatly expedited complex laparoscopic surgery and gastric operations are no exception. Special devices are now available. The advantages of this system including unique dressings that equilibrates to the intra-abdominal pressure, a good reach for the hand within the peritoneal cavity and easy insertion and removal of hands, swabs, and instrument to and from the peritoneal cavity. The hand assisted device is also used for extraction of the specimen and when appropriate for the reconstruction of the alimentary canal.

Additional future prospects

Laparoscopic surgery is now officially part of all the surgeon standard training curriculum. The best example is the progressive reduction of operative time as the surgeon's experience increases. Therefore training will be of vital importance for the future development of laparoscopic surgery. Accordingly outpatient surgery has become more and more popular and applicable to larger and larger patient populations and has also been shown to be safe even for the high risk patients.

Without advanced technology laparoscopic surgery would never have been born and developed. Imaging techniques were and will be of outmost importance and coupled to that computer science which opens the way to a series of technical achievements, the development of which, partly independent of the subject treated, are expanding up an almost vertical trajectory.

The concept of telepresence surgery has also to be considered. One of its advantages is the fact that the robot movements are incomparably more precise than those of a human hand. Some of the procedures can be controlled by a pre-recorded computer program, while the surgeon only intervenes in case of unexpected difficulties. This is already possible during preoperative assessment which, thanks to CT-scans, MRI and 3D reconstruction allows to navigate with extreme accuracy within the human body. Researchers are currently on their way to transmit tactile sensations to the surgeons hands thus making it possible for him or her to assess tissue resistance and resilience. We are now entering the world of virtual reality. All this equipment is still at a more or less rudimentary stage of research and development but prototypes are already in operation. Cholecystectomies and vascular sutures have already been performed in animal settings but we can predict a rapid development within this field. One area which probably is very suitable for telepresence is for instance hip replacement which is a very standardised procedure and the robot movements can be precisely defined in relation to fixed anatomical structures.

The most immediate implementation of these new technologies is their possible use for surgical training. Although abdominal viscera anatomy is quite difficult to reproduce by a computer programming, surgical simulators similar to the flight simulators used for pilot training are already made available to surgeons in some surgical centres. In the future they will probably take the place of training on live animals. This technology will also make it possible to altogether wipe out or at least considerably reduce the mediocre clinical results obtained at the beginning of the learning curve.

Neither our universities nor our hospitals taken individually, with their chronic financial difficulties are capable of setting up institutions which integrate high technologies requiring huge monitarian investments and interdisciplinary staff and researchers. The solution lies probably in contracts that will more firmly being together manufacturing firms, universities, hospitals of both private and community based systems.

Key references

- Bhutani MS. Interventional endoscopic ultrasonography: State of the art at the new millenium. *Endoscopy* 2000; 32: 62-71.
- Chae FH, Stiegmann GV. Current laparoscopic gastrointestinal surgery. Gastrointestinal. *Endoscopy* 1998; 47: 500-11.
- Conlon KC, *et al.* The value of minimal access surgery in the staging of patients with potentially resectable peripancreatic malignancy. *Ann Surg* 1996; 223: 134-40.
- Cuschieri A. Minimally invasive surgery: Hepatobiliary-pancreatic and forgut. *Endoscopy* 2000; 32: 331-44.
- Krummel TM. Surgical simulation and virtual reality: The coming revolution. *Ann Surg* 1998; 28: 635-7.
- Lambert R. Role of endoscopy in the prevention of digestive cancer: Application to colorectal cancer. *Endoscopy* 1998; 30: 628-40.
- Voitk AJ, *et al.* Is outpatient surgery safe for the higher risk patients ? *J Gastrointest Surg* 1998; 2: 156-8.

Novel approaches in the treatment of gastrointestinal and liver disease: a look into the future.
Galmiche J.P., ed. John Libbey Eurotext, Paris © 2000, pp. 77-86.

Intestinal transplantation

Olivier Goulet, Dominique Jan

Groupe de Transplantation Intestinale, Hôpital Necker-Enfants Malades, Paris, France

Small bowel transplantation (SBTx) was first demonstrated to be technically feasible in animals from 1902 and in humans in the early sixties [1]. The initial excitement however, rapidly decreased when posttransplant rejection and septicemia resulted in high morbidity and mortality. At the same time parenteral nutrition (PN) became a standard therapy for patients with intestinal dysfunction that allowed many adults and children to survive with a reasonable quality of life. Since its introduction, PN has improved greatly, especially with the development of home PN [2, 3]. However, long term PN is associated with complications such as liver impairment, bone disease, vascular thrombosis and sepsis that require innovative therapeutic modalities.

Intestinal transplantation (ITx) might become the alternative to definitive PN in patients with permanent intestinal failure. Indeed recent advances in immunosuppressive therapy and better monitoring as well as control of acute rejection have brought ITx into the realm of standard treatment of intestinal failure (IF). However this procedure may be performed in adult or pediatric patient under certain conditions. This short review focuses on current clinical results and indications of ITx and discuss the strategy regarding this challenging procedure.

In the 1980s, Cyclosporine A (CyA) did not allow, except in one child [4], long-term survival of adult or pediatric patients after isolated SBTx as it did after heart or liver transplantation. Two recent advances have made SBTx a promising option for the treatment of end-stage IF: combination with liver transplantation [5], and the development of FK 506 (tacrolimus) in the early 1990s [6]. The encouraging recent results indicate that ITx is becoming an acceptable clinical modality. However several questions remain: definition of IF, indications for ITx, type of transplantation isolated or combined liver-SBTx, patient selection and preparation, quality of life after transplantation.

Current clinical results after intestinal transplantation

Until now more than 500 ITx have been performed throught the world, essentially in the USA, Canada, France and UK. A previous report summarized the data of the Intestinal Transplant Registry including 49 patients treated with CyA [7].

Currently, the registry followed up 273 transplantations in 260 patients among 33 ITx programs [8]. Approximately two-thirds of recipients were children or adolescents. The transplants involved the isolated SB (SBTx) with or without the colon (41%), the liver + SB (LSBTx) (48%) and multivisceral (MTVTx) grafts (11%), including the stomach, pancreas, liver and SB. The main indications in the 154 children were short-bowel syndrome (67%), chronic intestinal pseudo-obstruction syndrome (10%), severe intractable diarrhea (6%), aganglionosis/Hirschsprung disease (6%) and in 106 adults: ischemia (21%), Crohn's disease (17%), trauma (15%), desmoid tumor (13%) or cancer (13%). The main immunosuppression included tacrolimus for 212 grafts (78%), cyclosporine A for 51 grafts (19%), and other or no immunosuppression for 8 grafts from living related donors (3%).

Overall patient survival was 58% for SBTx, 42% for combined LSBTx and 40% for MTVTx Death was due mainly to infections (47%), multiorgan failure (26%) or lymphoma (10%); Full nutrition autonomy with complete discontinuation of PN has been achieved in 77% of the cases and partial recovery was documented in another 14% giving total rehabilitation rate of 91% in survivors.

It is clear from the intestinal transplantation registry and from individual programs that prognosis improved during the last ten years. Patient survival is associated with the type of organ transplanted with better survival after SBTx. Nevertheless, interpretation of these results must be carefull as they represent the first 12 years' experience of a large number of programs in children and adults, using different immunosuppressive regimen. The results from the largest of these centers reflect the current situation more closely. In addition, programs that had performed at least 10 transplants have better graft and patient survival compared to programs that had performed less than 10 transplants [8].

Twenty-six pediatric transplants, 17 LSBTx and 9 SBTx, were reported by the University of Nebraska, who obtained patient survival rates of 73% and 100%, respectively, at one year [9]. Ninety-eight consecutive patients (59 children, 39 adults) received 104 allografts under tacrolimus-based immunosuppression: SBTx (n=37), LSBTx (n=50) or MTVTx (n=17). With a mean followup of 32 ± 26 months (range 1-86 months), 47 patients (48%) are alive with grafts that provide full (91%) or partial (9%) nutrition. Actuarial patient survival at 1 and 5 years (72% and 48%, respectively) was similar watever the type of graft [10]. Specific results concern 55 children having received 58 intestinal transplantation under tacrolimus/steroids immunosuppression [11]. They included SBTx (n=17), LSBTx (n=33) and MTVTx (n=8). The actuarial patient and primary graft survival rates at 1, 3, and 5 years are 72%, 55% and 55% for patient, and 66%, 48%, and 48% for graft, respectively. Thirty-one children have received 29 intestinal transplantation under tacrolimus/steroids immunosuppression, in Paris from November 1994, including SBTx (n=12), LSBTx (n=19). With 3 to 66 months followup, actuarial patient and primary graft survival rates are 70%, 83% for patient, and 30%, 83% for graft, respectively. Preliminary results have been recently published [12].

From the Registry as well as from the largest centres, it is currently difficult to analyze difference in survival rate between isolated and combined liver intestinal transplantation. In general, clinical status of liver-small bowel recipients is poor at the time of transplantation as suggested by the 1 and 2 year survival of patients who have not undergone transplantation being 30% and 22%, respectively [11] or the number of death on a waiting list [13]. On the other hand, the isolated SB graft not only has the highest incidence of rejection, but also require more intense immunosuppression to control it. This supports previous observations that simultaneous liver grafting may reduce the risk of intestinal rejection and experimental data [14]. The bone marrow augmentation trials do not provide improvement of patient or graft survival in pediatric or adult patient.

Complications after intestinal transplantation

In human, despite the presence of circulating donor-derived lymphocytes during the first few weeks after transplantation, clinical signs of graft *versus* host disease (GVHD) have rarely been reported. GVHD is not therefore a complication after intestinal transplantation as is graft rejection.

Intestinal allograft rejection remains the major complication after intestinal transplantation. Consequent to increased immunosuppression, graft rejection may further precipitate opportunistic infections that become additive factors in patient and graft losses. As rejection can occur rapidly and be life-threatening, close monitoring is required. This has led to the development of numerous diagnostic methods, which have not been validated in human intestinal transplantation or have limited value [15]. Hence regular biopsies of the proximal and distal ends of the graft for histologic or immunohistochemical analysis, are required [16, 18]. Clinical signs of rejection occurr later than histological and immunohistochemical signs and correspond to a relatively advanced rejection process with marked histological lesions. In addition, clinical manifestations are non specific markers of rejection. Thus, it is of importance to differentiate other sources of potential intestinal allograft disease that may clinically mimic rejection such as post-transplant lymphoproliferative disease (PTLD), Epstein-Barr virus (EBV), cytomegalovirus (CMV) or other bacterial/viral enterititis. Rejection and sepsis can be intimately related following SBTx when rejection compromises normal intestinal barrier mechanisms and bacterial translocation results with consequent multiorgan failure.

Viral infections are frequent such as CMV primo-infection or reactivation which is not always prevented by the use of preemptive treatment. Diagnosis of CMV infection improved with the use of polymerase chain reaction (PCR) shown as a sensitive method for the early detection of CMV infection in solid organ and intestinal graft recipients [19]. The incidence of CMV infection has been reported as reaching 29% of pediatric recipients of intestinal grafts [19]. It is recommended to avoid using a seropositive graft in a seronegative recipient. Nevertheless, patients who are awaiting composite grafts are frequently too sick to await a CMV-seronegative donor. CMV prophylaxis is now well established with wide use of gancyclovir.

EBV infection in association with immunosuppressive drugs used for solid organ transplantation can produce a spectrum of illness. A high incidence of EBV-induced PTLD has been reported. The incidence increases with the degree of immunosuppression. Quantitative EBV-PCR in the peripheral blood has recently allowed for early diagnosis as well as follow-up of patients with EBV infection. This may allow the diagnoses of EBV infection before the development of PTLD. In the case of established EBV-related PTLD, therapeutic changes based on quantitative PCR and use of monoclonal antibodies directed against B-cells are helpful in preventing the end phases of this disease. Donor selection and prevention of EBV infection are unsolved problems.

Other severe life-threatening complications have been reported such as diffuse adenovirus enterocolitis or hemophagocytosis. Early identification of viral infections, based on the repeated use of appropriate methods, may help avoiding the misdiagnosis of rejection leading to an unecessary increase of immunosuppressive treatment with consequent excacerbation of the underlying infections condition.

Graft function

Factors, such as denervation, lymphatic disruption, ischemia-reperfusion, immunosuppressive treatment, rejection and infection may explain impaired function of the intestinal graft [20]. Studies performed in animals have shown that intestinal transplantation disturbs the absorption of carbohydrates, lipids, glutamine, water and electrolytes. Intestinal motility may be severely impaired due to the loss of extrinsic innervation of the small bowel, ischemia reperfusion and/or immunological activation [21].

Feeding must resume as early as possible, either by mouth, or by an enteral tube, as this ensures optimal mucosal trophicity and reduces gastrointestinal stasis, which is a source of intraluminal bacterial overgrowth. Clinical experience demonstrate that because of water-electrolytes malabsorption and abnormal motility, normal intestinal transit and stool volume may require several weeks to be achieved. If the recipient has no colon, combined small-large bowel transplantation has physiological advantages in terms of water and electrolyte reabsorption, slowing of intestinal transit and trophic factors, through colonic synthesis of short-chain fatty acids.

Finally, it is currently considered that intestinal transplantation restores an enteral axis capable of ensuring digestion and absorption, and that full function allow PN to be withdrawn completely.

Indications for intestinal transplantation

Short bowel syndrome caused by extensive resection of the small bowel, has been logically the first indication for intestinal transplantation. After extensive resection of the small bowel, most neonates now survive and acquire gastrointestinal autonomy after a period depending on extent and site of resection, and the persistence of disease in the remaining gut [22]. Only, a small number of children (approximately 10 to 15%) do not acquire gastrointestinal autonomy even after several years [23]. In older children or adolescents, after extensive intestinal resection, intestinal adaptation, and intestinal absorption sufficient to meet growth requirements, can only be obtained if the length of remaining small bowel is more than 40 cm beyond the angle of Treitz. Some children do not become autonomous even after more than 10 years of home-based PN, and are thus candidates for intestinal transplantation.

In all these short small bowel conditions, transplantation can only be envisaged once it has been formally shown that the remnant bowel cannot adapt. Surgical approach such as lengthening of the small bowel, loop interposition or assembly of a « reverse » intestinal loop have to be attempted [24, 25]. Trophic factors such as recombinant human growth hormone (rhGH), will probably contribute to decrease the need for intestinal transplantation in the near future. Clinical studies have provided controversial results [26, 27]. Open trial in pediatric and adult patients are still in process in the USA and in France.

Apart from these purely anatomical indications, intestinal transplantation can also be indicated in children with motility disorders or mucosal disease. Motility disorders include extensive Hirschsprung disease (HD) and chronic intestinal pseudoobstruction syndrome (CIPOS). The first one raises the same problems than SBS with two mains differences. The non functionning colon is excluded and the HD free small bowel has motility disorders. Thus when normally inervated small bowel is shorter than 60 cm the probability for long-term PN dependency is high. Logically this situation requires a combined colon transplantation. CIPOS is a very heterogeneous condition in terms of clinical presentation, associated uropathy, histopathologic features, severity of motility disorders and outcome. In our experience 20 to 25% of patients will become definitively dependent on PN [28].

Two mucosal disease responsible for permanent intestinal failure are currently recognized as requiring intestinal transplantation: Microvillous inclusion disease (MID) and epithelial dysplasia (ED). Both are inherited disorders with neonatal, onset of severe watery diarrhea. MID involve the intracellular pathway of brushborder development while ED is associated with abnormal enterocytes and basement membrane. For both the primary defect is currently not known. Children with one of these two mucosal disease underwent successfull SBTx isolated or in combination with liver [29, 30].

In adults, the main indications for intestinal transplantation is an inadaptable very short small bowel after subtotal or total resection. This is secondary to vascular, mechanical, traumatic or atheromatous events, leading to necrosis of whole or part of the small bowel. Tumors and infiltration of the mesentery (*e.g.* Gardner's syndrome) and the sequelae of radiation enteritis or chronic intestinal pseudo-obstruction syndrome are also indications for intestinal transplantation in adults [31]. Crohn's disease extending to the small bowel is a case apart, although transplants have been done in this context. Crohn's disease raises the problem of relapse on the graft as it was recently reported [32].

Strategy for intestinal transplantation

The number of potential candidates for intestinal transplantation was evaluated in a British study at 2 per year per million inhabitants, a figure that includes both adults and children being on home-PN at the time of the study [33]. Indeed, intestinal transplantation is theoretically indicated for all patients permanently dependent on PN. Intestinal transplantation is possible and is, in some conditions, the logical therapeutic option. Functional grafts lead to gastrointestinal autonomy (weaning of PN) while maintaining satisfactory nutritional status and normal growth in childhood. However, as PN is generally well tolerated, even for long periods, each indication for transplantation must be carefully weighed up in terms of survival rate, morbidity and quality of life. By excluding malignant disease and immune deficiency, survival rates of patients with chronic intestinal failure on long-term home PN remain higher than after intestinal transplantation [2, 3]. Intestinal transplantation is often accompanied with numerous life-threatening complications as those briefly reviewed above, leading to recurrent and/or long term hospitalization and some times poor outcome. Evaluation of quality of life after intestinal transplantation among home PN was recently performed in adult patients using Quality of life instrument in the form of a self-administered questionnaire [34]. Intestinal transplant recipients with functioning grafts reported significant improvement in the quality of their life and function. This information is encouraging and should be used toward future advancement in intestinal transplantation.

However, even with the most optimistic interpretation of available data, when long-term PN is effective and well-tolerated, it can be used pending further progress in intestinal transplantation. In contrast, when PN has reached its limits, especially those associated with extensive thrombosis, recurrent sepsis, severe metabolic disorders or advanced liver disease, intestinal transplantation must be undertaken.

Intestinal transplantation: isolated or combined with liver

Patients with irreversible intestinal failure and end-stage liver disease are undoubtly candidate for a life saving procedure such as combined liver small bowel transplantation (LSBTx). Patients with severe hepatic fibrosis or cirrhosis are more difficult to manage. Repeated liver biopsie within 6 to 12 months and careful assessment for portal hypertension are mandatory. It is difficult to predict the liver damage related to persistent need for PN or to rejection and/or infection during the first weeks or months following transplantation. In addition, it is difficult to assess the amount of functioning liver necessary to withstand the insult of portal diversion during transplantation procedure. Thus those patients with severe hepatic fibrosis or cirrhosis are usually listed for LSBTx.

Patients with irreversible intestinal failure and PN dependency without consistent liver disease must satisfy rigorous criteria to be considered as candidates for isolated SBTx. They must fulfill at least one of the following criteria: extensive thrombosis imperiling the ability to administer PN, recurrent life-threatening sepsis, severe metabolic disorders avoiding to met nutritional requirements with consequent failure to thrive in children, underlying disease with high water-electrolytes losses with risk of life-threatening dehydratation in case of PN disruption.

Timing for referral

Two main reason lead currently to delayed timing of referral. First, criteria for either small bowel or combined liver-small bowel transplantation continue to be debated. Secondly few centre use to manage all the stage of intestinal failure from onset to ITx, including home PN program. In a recent study, the mortality rate, death within 6 months of evaluation for transplantation was 90% in children with short gut, 50% in those with mucosal disease and 40% with CIPOS [20]. Factors impacting the survival of children with intestinal failure referred for intestinal transplantation have been studied in a serie of 257 patients (mean age, 3.4 ± 0.26 years) evaluated for Itx [35]. Only 82 (32%) underwent ITx (68 LSBTx) with a mean waiting time of 10.1 ± 1.3 months. Of the 175 patients who were not transplanted, 120 died. The main factors associated with poor prognosis were: age $\leq$ 1 year, surgical disease, bridging fibrosis or cirrhosis, bilirubin levels > 3 mg/dl, thrombocytopenia.

In our experience time to go from portal fibrosis to cirrhosis in around 12 months similar to waiting time [36]. Once cirrhosis has been established, survival at 1 year is only 30% [35]. It is well established that patients referred for combined small bowel liver transplantation are more debilitated, have multiple complications, and have prolonged stays in intensive care unit. It may explain the lower patient and graft survival rate according to isolated SBTx reported from several programs [9, 11]. It was suggested that early isolated SBTx with such a short period of postoperative hospitalization could well prove to be cost-effective compared with the intensive use of resources that characterizes the short bowel patient with liver failure.

Finally, since pediatric patients represent almost two-third of indication for small bowel transplantation, appropriate therapeutic strategies should be developed. It is first required to recognize as early, as possible the patient with irreversible IF such as extreme short bowel syndrome, or congenital disease of intestinal mucosa. These patients should be referred early to multidisciplinary teams involved in small bowel transplantation in optimal nutritional status. Beath et al have reported a marked discrepancy in clinical status between children referred for ITx from centers with and without nutritional care teams. Indeed, adequate PN intake, early cyclic PN, use of enteral feeding and ursodeoxycholic are mandatory. It is also essential to have appropriate policies in the management of central line to avoid sepsis and thrombosis [37].

For the other patients dependent on long term PN and who faile to adapt after extensive small bowel resection or because intestinal pseudo-obstruction syndrome, prevention of PN related complication and careful monitoring should allow to perform isolated small bowel transplantation instead of a life saving procedure such as combined SB liver transplantation. Thus patient selection require precise criteria for diagnosing irreversible intestinal failure and early referral for assessment and transplantation.

Particular procedures

Living related donors

Intestinal grafts are usually obtained from size matched brain-dead adults or children. ABO identity is necessary to avoid hemolysis related to circulating antibodies. It is difficult to obtain HLA compatibility, mainly for logistic reasons (the graft poorly tolerates ischemia). However, the longest survival time before the advent of CsA was observed after intrafamilial transplantation. Long survival times have since been obtained in intrafamilial transplantation with CsA or FK506 immunosuppression [38] and without immunosuppression in one case of identical twins [38].

Reduced sized composite liver-intestinal allograft

Strict donor selection to prevent factors that may adversely affect the intestinal graft and size matching have limited donor availability. These factors contribute to the long waiting time for pediatric patients. Reduced-sized orthotopic composite liver-intestinal allografts are technically feasible and may increase the donor pool [40, 41].

Multivisceral transplantation

"Cluster" transplantation of organs from the celiac region (liver, stomach, duodenum-pancreas and small bowel) was reported for the first time in 1989 [42]. It now represents 16% of all intestinal grafts. This procedure raises specific technical problems, but immunosuppressive treatment is not different. Multiorgan transplants are only envisaged, especially in adults, if necessitated by anatomical considerations, such as a tumor invading the celiac region.

Finally, intestinal transplantation requires a strategy based on a long-term management by a multidisciplinary team aiming to demonstrate the irreversibility of intestinal failure, to avoid complications of long-term parenteral nutrition. Candidates for intestinal transplantation should be assessed early and transplanted as early if needed in order to avoid death on waiting list or morbidity after transplantation.

References

1. Schraut W. Current status of small bowel transplantation. *Gastroenterology* 1988; 94: 525-35.
2. Colomb V, Goulet O, Ricour C. Home enteral and parenteral nutrition. Baillère's Clinical *Gastroenterology* 1998; 12: 877-94.
3. Messing B, Lemann M, Landais P, Gouttebel MC, Gérard-Boncompain M, Saudin F, *et al*. Prognosis of patients with chronic intestinal failure receiving long-term home parenteral nutrition in France and Belgium. *Gastroenterology* 1995; 108: 1005-10.
4. Goulet O, Révillon Y, Brousse N, Jan D, Canioni D, Rambaud C, *et al*. Successsful small bowel transplantation in an infant. *Transplantation* 1992; 53: 940-3.
5. Grant D, Wall W, Mimerault R, Zhong R, Ghent C, Garcia B, *et al*. Successful small bowel-liver transplantation. *Lancet* 1990; 335: 181-4.

6. Todo S, Tsakis A, Abu-Elmagd K,, Reyes J, Fung JJ, Casavilla A, *et al.* Cadaveric small bowel and small bowel-liver transplantation in humans. *Transplantation* 1992; 53: 369-76.
7. Grant D. Intestinal Transplantation Registry on behalf of the Current results of intestinal transplantation. *Lancet* 1996; 347: 1801-3.
8. Grant D. Intestinal transplantation: 1997 Report of the International Registry. *Transplantation* 1999; 15: 1061-4.
9. Langnas AN, Shaw BW, Antonson DL, Kaufman SS, Mack DR, Heffron TG, Fox IJ, Vanderhoof JA. Preliminary experience with intestinal transplantation in infants and children. *Pediatrics* 1996; 97: 443-8.
10. Abu-Elmagd K, Reyes J, Todo S, Rao A, Lee R, Irish W, *et al.* Clinical intestinal transplantation: new perspectives and immunologic considerations. *J Am Coll Surg* 1998; 186: 512-25.
11. Reyes J, Bueno J, Kocoshis S, Green M, Abu-Elmagd K, Furukawa H, *et al.* Current Status of Intestinal Transplantation in Children. *J Pediatr Surg* 1998; 243-54.
12. Goulet O, Jan D, Lacaille F, Colomb V, Michel JL, Damotte D *et al.* Intestinal transplantation in children: Preliminary experience in Paris. *J Parenter Ent Nutr* 1999; 23: S121-5.
13. Beath SV, Brook GA, Kelly DA, Buckels SAC, Mayer AD. Demand for pediatric small bowel transplantation in the United Kingdom. *Transplant Proc* 1998; 30: 2531-2.
14. Sarnacki S, Révillon Y, Cerf-Bensussan N, Calise D, Goulet O, Brousse N. Long term small bowel graft survival induced by spontaneously tolerated liver allograft in inbred rat strains. *Transplantation* 1992; 54: 383-5.
15. Goulet O. Recent studies on small intestinal transplantation. *Gastroenterology* 1997; 13: 500-9.
16. Lee RG, Nakamura K, Tsamandas AC, Abu-Elmagd K, Furukawa H, Hudson WR, *et al.* Pathology of human intestinal transplantation. *Gastroenterology* 1996; 110: 1820-34.
17. Goulet O, Brousse N, Révillon Y, Ricour C. Pathology of human intestinal transplantation. In: Grant D, Wood RFM, eds. Small bowel transplantation. Edward Arnold: London 1993: 112-20.
18. Tzakis A, Thompson JF. Current status of diagnosis of small bowel rejection. *Pediat Transplant* 1998; 2: 87-8.
19. Green M, Bueno J, Sigurdsson L, *et al.* Unique aspects of the infection complications of intestinal transplantation. *Curr Op Org Transplant.* 1999; 4: 361-7.
20. Kim J, Fryer J, Craig RM. Absorptive function following small intestinal transplantation. *Dig Dis Sci* 1998; 43: 1925-30.
21. Kusunoki M, Ishii H, Nakao K, Fujiwara Y, Yamamura T, Utsonomiya J. Long-Term effects of small bowel transplantation on intestinal motility. *Transplantation* 1995; 60: 897-9.
22. Goulet O, Révillon Y, Jan D, Jan D, De Potter S, Maurage C, Lortat-Jacob S, Martelli H, Nihoul-Fekete C, Ricour C. Neonatal short bowel syndrome. *J Pediatr* 1991; 119: 18-23.
23. Goulet O, Révillon Y, Jan D, De Potter S, Colomb V, Sadoun E, BenHariz M, Ricour C. Which patients need small bowel transplantation for neonatal short bowel syndrome. *Transplant Proc* 1992; 24: 1058-9.
24. Thompson JS, Langnas AN, Pinch LW, Kaufman S, Shaw BW, Vanderhoof J, *et al.* Surgical approach to short-bowel syndrome. Experience in a population of 160 patients. *Ann Surg* 1995; 222: 600-5.
25. Panis Y, Messing B, Rivet P, Coffin B, Hautefeuille P, Matuchansky C, *et al.* Segmental reversal of the small bowel as an alternative to intestinal transplantation in patients with short bowel syndrome. *Ann Surg* 1997; 225: 401-7.
26. Byrne TA, Persinger RL, Young LS, Ziegler TR, Wilmore DW. A new treatment for patients with short-bowel syndrome: growth hormone, glutamine and a modified diet. *Ann Surg* 1995; 22: 243-55.
27. Scolapio JS, Camilleri M, Fleming CR, Vonne Oenning LA, Burton DD, Sebo TJ, *et al.* Effect of growth hormone, glutamine, and diet on adaptation in short-bowel syndrome: a randomized, controlled study. *Gastroenterology* 1997; 113: 1074-81.

28. Goulet O, Jobert-Giraud A, Michel JL, Jaubert F, Lortat-Jacob S, Colomb V, *et al.* Chronic intestinal pseudoobstruction syndrome in pediatric patients. *Eur J Pediatr Surg* 1999 (in press).
29. Oliva MM, Perman JA, Saavedra JM, Young-Ramsaran J, Schwartz KB. Successful intestinal transplantation for microvillous inclusion disease. *Gastroenterology* 1994; 106: 771-4.
30. Lacaille F, Cuenod B, Colomb V, Jan D, Canioni D, Revillon Y, Ricour C, Goulet O. Combined liver and smal bowel transplantation in a child with epithelial dysplasia. *J Pediatr Gastroenterol Nutr* 1998; 27: 230-3.
31. Asfar S, Zhong R, Grant DR. Small Bowel Transplantation. *Surg Clin North Am* 1994; 74: 1197-210.
32. Sustendo-Reodica N, Ruiz P, Rogers A, Viciana Al, OConn H, Tzakis AG. Recurrent Crohn's disease in transplanted bowel. *Lancet* 1997; 349: 688-91.
33. Clark I, Lear PA, Wood S, Lennard-Jones JE, Wood RFM. Potential candidates for small bowel transplantation. *Br Med Surg* 1992; 79: 676-9.
34. Rovera GM, Di Martini A, Schoen RE, Rakela J, Abu-Elmagd, Graham TO. Quality of life of patients after intestinal transplantation. *Transplantation* 1998; 66: 1141-5.
35. Bueno J, Ohwada S, Kocoshis S, Mazariegos GV, Dvorchik I, Sigurdsson L, Di Lorenzo C, Abu-Elmagd K, Reyes J. Factors impacting the survival of chidren with intestinal failure referred for intestinal transplantation. *J Pediatr Surg* 1999; 34: 27-33.
36. Colomb V, Jobert A, Lacaille F, Fournet JC, Ricour C, Jan D, Revillon Y, Goulet O. Parenteral nutrition associated liver disease in children: natural history and prognosis. *J Pediatr Gastroenterol Nutr* 2000, in press.
37. Goulet O. Intestinal failure in children. *Transplant Proc* 1998; 30: 2523-5.
38. Fujimoto Y, Uemoto S, Inomata Y, Kurokawa T, Koshiba T, Takatsuki M, Hino H, Tanaka K. Living-related small bowel transplant: management of rejection and infection. *Transplant Proc* 1998; 30: 1149.
39. Morel P, Kadry Z, Charbonnet P, Bednarkiewicz M, Faiduth B. Paediatric living related intestinal transplantation between two monozygotic twins: a 1-year follow-up. *Lancet* 2000; 355: 723-4.
40. Reyes J, Fishbein T, Bueno J, Mazariegos G, Abu-Elmagd K. Reduced-size orthotopic composite liver-intestinal allograft. *Transplantation* 1998; 66: 489-92.
41. Bueno J, Abu-Elmagd K, Mazariegos G, Madariaga J, Fun Reyes J. Composite liver small bowel allografts with preservation donor duodenum and hepatic biliary system in children. *J Pediatr Surg* 2000; 35: 291-5.
42. Starzl TE, Rowe MI, Todo S. Transplantation of multiple abdominal viscera. *JAMA* 1989; 261: 1449-57.

New developments in abdominal imaging

Guido N.J. Tytgat

Academic Medical Center, Department of Gastroenterology and Hepatology, Amsterdam, The Netherlands

New developments in abdominal imaging relate to intraductal ultrasonography (IDUS), auto-fluorescence technology and computer tomography colonography (CTC).

Intraductal ultrasonography

Advances in ultrasound technology led to miniaturisation of the ultrasound transducers. This resulted in the development of high-frequency miniprobes which allowed for passage through the instrumentation channel of endoscopes. Currently IDUS is the most sensitive imaging technique for visualisation of the biliary and pancreatic ductal system.

With 20MHz ultrasound frequencies the normal bile duct consists of an inner hypoechoic layer, corresponding to fibromuscular tissue and perimuscular loose connective tissue, and a hyperechoic outer layer corresponding to subserosal fat tissue [1]. It is not possible to reliably differentiate T1-bile duct tumours (no infiltration through the fibromuscular layer) from T2-tumours (penetration through the fibromuscular layer). In patients who had an endoprosthesis *in situ* for 2-5 weeks, the wall is significantly thicker with a mean thickness of 2-2.5 mm [2].

The two most important indications for intraductal ultrasound of the biliary system are characterisation of biliary strictures and locoregional tumour staging of cholangiocarcinomas and ampullary tumours. IDUS can be used to characterize bile duct strictures, differentiating benign from malignant stenosis [3], but Gress *et al.* studied the IDUS characteristics of 36 patients with bile duct strictures and could not identify any obvious differences between benign and malignant lesions [4]. Therefore IDUS cannot reliably distinguish benign from malignant biliary stenosis. It should not be used as a substitute for true histological or cytological investigation. IDUS may, however, be a valuable tool in the staging of biliary and ampullary tumours.

Compared to EUS, IDUS has three important technical advantages in staging these tumours. Firstly, IDUS can be performed in the same endoscopic session as the ERCP, whereas EUS requires an additional procedure, Secondly, IDUS does not require a water-filled balloon for acoustic coupling that may compress small ampullary tumours. Thirdly, in IDUS the scanning plane of the probe is perpendicular to the axis of the distal common bile duct, whereas tangential imaging is almost inevitable in EUS.

The high accuracy of IDUS in staging small ampullary tumours, resulting from its excellent differentiation between the sphincter of Oddi and the duodenal wall, may thus identify those patients in whom local resection, such as local surgical resection or endoscopic papillectomy, is sufficient for radical resection.

IDUS may also play a role in diagnosing mucin-producing tumours of the pancreas. These tumours, which may be (pre)malignant, are difficult to visualize with standard imaging modalities [5].

The high sensitivity of IDUS in visualizing small pancreatic lesions may also be useful in the diagnosis of pancreatic neuroendocrine tumours that had standard EUS [5].

Although IDUS is currently still in its infancy, exciting technical developments await the future. Three-dimensional intraductal ultrasound is already being developed and may allow for even more detailed visualization of the relationship of tumours and their direct surroundings. Combining IDUS with intravascular ultrasound (IVUS) may increase the sensitivity in discovering tumour ingrowth. IDUS may play a role in targeting local treatment of tumours, *e.g.* with intraluminal brachytherapy or photodynamic therapy, as well as in the assessment of treatment response.

Autofluorescence imaging

Reflectance spectroscopy, elastic scattering spectroscopy, optical coherence tomography (OCT), raman spectroscopy, and fluorescence spectroscopy are amongst the optical techniques that can be used to diagnose tissue *in vivo* [6]. These techniques all exploit distinct microarchitectural and biochemical changes in tissue.

There are two approaches to fluorescence detection of dysplasia [7]. One approach is to use tissue autofluorescence, *i.e.* the fluorescence originating from naturally occurring endogenous fluorophores that are specific to normal or dysplastic tissue. Another approach is to use induced fluorescence by administering exogenous fluorophores that tend to accumulate preferentially in malignant transformed tissue [8]. Most of these exogenous fluorescent agents, however, have an associated photodynamic effect limiting their use for mass screening purposes. The two applicable autofluorescence techniques are fluorescence spectroscopy (optical biopsy) and fluorescence imaging.

In Laser Induced Fluorescence Spectroscopy (LIFS) a laser is used to generate monochromatic light. The light source is coupled to a small diameter fiberoptic probe. By advancing the probe through the instrument channel of the endoscope it is placed in contact with the mucosa.

In Laser Induced Fluorescence Spectroscopy (LIFS) a laser is used to generate monochromatic light. The light source is coupled to a small diameter fiberoptic probe. By advancing the probe through the instrument channel of the endoscope it is placed in contact with the mucosa. The optical probe is used to both excite and detect the tissue fluorescence. Since only a small volume of tissue (2-4 mm^2) is sampled at a time, the technique is also called optical biopsy.

From a clinical perspective, however, probing a large surface area of intestinal mucosa with point spectroscopy is rather cumbersome. A fluorescence imaging system incorporated in a standard endoscope would enable screening of large surface areas of mucosa, detection of occult lesions and targeted biopsy sampling. By illuminating the entire endoscopic field of view with excitation light, fluorescence images can be collected in parallel with the standard endoscopic image.

Light Induced Fluorescence Endoscopy (LIFE) is a similar ratio fluorescence imaging technique for the gastrointestinal tract. The LIFE system uses a narrow-hand blue light source in conjunction with a standard fiberoptic endoscope and a dual amplified CCD camera. Using this setup, dysplastic lesions occult to standard endoscopy have been visualized [9, 10].

On a selected group of 80 patients with Barrett's esophagus, areas of high-grade dysplasia and early carcinoma could be detected with a sensitivity and a specificity of 87% [10], but only 4 of 22 areas of low-grade dysplasia could be identified.

The feasibility to surpass the naked eye by detecting otherwise endoscopically undetectable neoplastic lesions has already been established. Double-ration fluorescence algorithms, time-resolved fluorescence detection and combinations with other optical techniques are soon to be implemented.

Computed tomography colonography

Currently, CTC still requires a dry and clean colon and therefore standard oral preparation as for colonoscopy is necessary. The colon is insufflated with approximately 2 L of room air or carbon dioxide gas. For optimal CT-imaging, the colon should be fully distended without filling of small bowel loops. To minimize motion artefacts, a spasmolytic agent (*e.g.* scopolamine, 20 mg) is administered intravenously just prior to data acquisition. Subsequently the abdomen is scanned in three to four 20-second breath holds using a helical CT-scanner. Data sets re obtained both in the prone and supine position to compensate for residual fluid in the colon. Because of the high contrast between the gas-filled colon and the soft tissue of the colonic wall, only a low-dose setting (70 mA) is necessary for adequate imaging [11]. The radiation dose of CTC is therefore relatively low.

Interpretation of CTC consists of viewing the non-reformatted axial CT images, reformatted two dimensional views, and three dimensional projections. When the three dimensional images are displayed sequentially in real-time (15-30 images/second) a simulated endoscopic view of the colon is created. The two-dimensional views are particularly useful for characterisation of lesions, *e.g.* retained stool can be discriminated from polyps due to the characteristic heterogeneous appearance on two-dimensional images. The three dimensional views are most effective in differentiating haustral folds from polyps and are probably more sensitive than other types of image display for detection of small lesions.

The development of stool markers may further improve the differentiation between retained stool and true polyps.

CTC detection rates of colonic polyps ≥ 8 mm in diameter are good, but not excellent. The majority of the incorrect diagnoses however are due to perceptive errors or poor colon preparation. Further improvement of the technique in the near future should be able to deal with most of these technical problems.

In the future it may however be possible to obtain CTC images with only minor preparation. The patient will then ingest a small amount of a contrast agent 24-48 hours prior to the investigation. This contrast agent will specifically label the stools which enables digital subtraction of faecal matter from the CT images.

Currently, image processing and interpretation is labour intensive, often requiring an excess of 45 minutes. Software is being developed that will allow for faster data processing and real-time interaction between the examiner and the date set. Computerized assessment of the colonic wall thickness may assist radiological interpretation and allow for examinations to be interpreted correctly within only a few minutes.

CTC is a new and exciting imaging technique for colonic lesions. In theory, CTC has all the characteristics that may make it the ideal screening tool for colorectal disease. Within five years CTC preparation may require only the ingestion of 100 ml of liquid stool marker two days prior to the procedure. CT scanning will be performed in a single breath hold after intra-venous administration of a spasmolytic agent and a mucosal contrast agent. While the patient is still on the CT table, the data set will be automatically processed and interpreted by the computer. The radiologist and/or endoscopist will immediately evaluate the results, interact with the data set and obtain additional images if necessary. The investigation will take less than 15 minutes and will be more cost-effective than barium enema or colonoscopy. CTC will have an excellent sensitivity and specificity for detecting even small colonic lesions. Since the entire length of the colon is visualized (including redundant colons) and the whole colonic surface is imaged (including "blind corners"), CTC will be superior to any other diagnostic modality of the colon, including colonoscopy. Diagnostic colonoscopy may well become obsolete and it will become increasingly important for gastroenterologists to receive adequate training in therapeutic endoscopy.

References

1. Tamada K, Kanai N, Ueno N, *et al.* Limitations of intraductal ultrasonography in differentiating between bile duct cancer in stage T1 and T2: *in vitro* and *in vivo* studies. *Endoscopy* 1997; 29: 721-5.
2. Tamada K, Tomiyama T, Ichiyama M, *et al.* Influence of biliary drainage catheter on bile duct wall thickness as measured by intraductal ultrasonography. *Gastrointest Endosc* 1998; 47: 28-32.
3. Tamada K Ueno N, Tomiyama T, *et al.* Characterization of biliary strictures using intra-ductal ultrasonography: comparison with percutaneous cholangioscopic biopsy. *Gastrointest Endosc* 1998; 47: 341-9.
4. Gress F, Chen YK, Sherman S, *et al.* Experience with a catheter-based ultrasound probe in the bile duct and pancreas. *Endoscopy* 1995; 27: 178-84.
5. Mukai H, Yasuda K, Nakajima M. Differential diagnosis of mucin-producing tumours of the pancreas by intraductal ultrasonography and peroral pancreatoscopy. *Endoscopy* 1998; 30 (Suppl. 1): A99: A102.
6. Barr H, Dix T, Stone N. Optical spectroscopy for the early diagnosis of gastrointestinal malignancy. *Laser Med Sci* 1998; 13: 3-13.
7. Haringsma J, Tytgat GNJ. Fluorescence and autofluorescence. *Baillière's Clinical Gastroenterol* 1999; 13: 1-10.
8. Stepp H, Sroka R, Baumgartner R. Fluorescence endoscopy of gastrointestinal diseases: basic principles, techniques, and clinical experience. *Endoscopy* 1998; 30: 379-86.
9. Haringsma J, Tytgat GNJ. Light-induced fluorescence endoscopy for the *in vivo* detection of colorectal dysplasia. *Gastroenterology* 1998; 114: A606.
10. Haringsma J, Prawirodirdjo W, Tytgat GNJ. Accuracy of fluorescence imaging of dysplasia in Barrett's esophagus. *Gastroenterology* 1999; 115: A418.
11. Hara AK, Johnson CD, Reed JE, *et al.* Reducing data size and radiation dose for CT colonography. *AJR* 1997; 168: 1181-4.

Achevé d'imprimer par Corlet, Imprimeur, S.A.
14110 Condé-sur-Noireau (France)
N° d'Imprimeur : 46629 - Dépôt légal : juin 2000
Imprimé en U.E.